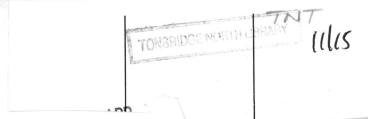

Dr Dawn Harper is a GP based in ⟨⟩ surgery in Stroud. She has been work⟨⟩ years. Dawn is best known as one of th⟨⟩ winning programme *Embarrassing Bodi*⟨⟩ ⟨⟩ries and last year celebrated its hundredth ⟨⟩ ...ons have included *Embarrassing Fat Bodies*, *Embarrassing Teen Bodies* and *Embarrassing Bodies: Live from the clinic*.

Dawn is the presenter of Channel 4's series *Born Naughty?*, one of the doctors on ITV1's *This Morning* and the resident GP on the health hour on LBC radio. She writes for a variety of publications, including *Healthspan* and *Healthy Food Guide*. Her first book, *Dr Dawn's Health Check*, was published by Mitchell Beazley. *Dr Dawn's Guide to Digestive Health* is one of five Dr Dawn Guides published by Sheldon Press in 2015. Dawn qualified at London University in 1987. When not working, she is a keen cyclist and an enthusiastic supporter of children's charities. Her website is at <www.drdawn.com>. Follow her on Twitter @drdawnharper.

Overcoming Common Problems Series

Selected titles

A full list of titles is available from Sheldon Press,
36 Causton Street, London SW1P 4ST and on our website at
www.sheldonpress.co.uk

Breast Cancer: Your treatment choices
Dr Terry Priestman

Chronic Fatigue Syndrome: What you need to know about CFS/ME
Dr Megan A. Arroll

Cider Vinegar
Margaret Hills

Coeliac Disease: What you need to know
Alex Gazzola

Coping Successfully with Hiatus Hernia
Dr Tom Smith

Coping with Difficult Families
Dr Jane McGregor and Tim McGregor

Coping with Epilepsy
Dr Pamela Crawford and Fiona Marshall

Coping with Memory Problems
Dr Sallie Baxendale

Coping with the Psychological Effects of Illness
Dr Fran Smith, Dr Carina Eriksen and Professor Robert Bor

Coping with Schizophrenia
Professor Kevin Gournay and Debbie Robson

Coping with Thyroid Disease
Mark Greener

Depressive Illness: The curse of the strong
Dr Tim Cantopher

Dr Dawn's Guide to Brain Health
Dr Dawn Harper

Dr Dawn's Guide to Heart Health
Dr Dawn Harper

Dr Dawn's Guide to Weight and Diabetes
Dr Dawn Harper

Dr Dawn's Guide to Women's Health
Dr Dawn Harper

The Empathy Trap: Understanding antisocial personalities
Dr Jane McGregor and Tim McGregor

The Fibromyalgia Healing Diet
Christine Craggs-Hinton

Fibromyalgia: Your treatment guide
Christine Craggs-Hinton

Helping Elderly Relatives
Jill Eckersley

The Holistic Health Handbook
Mark Greener

How to Stop Worrying
Dr Frank Tallis

Invisible Illness: Coping with misunderstood conditions
Dr Megan A. Arroll and Professor Christine P. Dancey

Living with the Challenges of Dementia: A guide for family and friends
Patrick McCurry

Living with Complicated Grief
Professor Craig A. White

Living with Fibromyalgia
Christine Craggs-Hinton

Living with Hearing Loss
Dr Don McFerran, Lucy Handscomb and Dr Cherilee Rutherford

Overcoming Fear with Mindfulness
Deborah Ward

Overcoming Low Self-esteem with Mindfulness
Deborah Ward

Overcoming Stress
Professor Robert Bor, Dr Carina Eriksen and Dr Sara Chaudry

Overcoming Worry and Anxiety
Dr Jerry Kennard

Physical Intelligence: How to take charge of your weight
Dr Tom Smith

Post-Traumatic Stress Disorder: Recovery after accident and disaster
Professor Kevin Gournay

The Self-Esteem Journal
Alison Waines

The Stroke Survival Guide
Mark Greener

Ten Steps to Positive Living
Dr Windy Dryden

Treating Arthritis: The drug-free way
Margaret Hills and Christine Horner

Understanding High Blood Pressure
Dr Shahid Aziz and Dr Zara Aziz

Understanding Yourself and Others: Practical ideas from the world of coaching
Bob Thomson

When Someone You Love Has Depression: A handbook for family and friends
Barbara Baker

Overcoming Common Problems

Dr Dawn's Guide to Digestive Health

DR DAWN HARPER

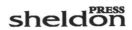

Dedicated to Sarah Eglin, Mark Downie and all the team at Maverick TV

Thank you for following your gut instinct and giving me some amazing opportunities

First published in Great Britain in 2015

Sheldon Press
36 Causton Street
London SW1P 4ST
www.sheldonpress.co.uk

British Library Cataloguing-in-Publication Data
A catalogue record for this book is available from the British Library

ISBN 978–1–84709–362–2
eBook ISBN 978–1–84709–363–9

Typeset by Fakenham Prepress Solutions, Fakenham, Norfolk NR21 8NN
First printed in Great Britain by Ashford Colour Press
Subsequently digitally reprinted in Great Britain

eBook by Fakenham Prepress Solutions, Fakenham, Norfolk NR21 8NN

Produced on paper from sustainable forests

Contents

Note to the reader

This is not a medical book and is not intended to replace advice from your doctor. Consult your pharmacist or doctor if you believe you have any of the symptoms described, and if you think you might need medical help.

1

Anatomy and function of the digestive tract

Our digestive system is effectively a long muscular tube starting at the mouth and ending at the anus; in adults this is about seven to nine metres long. I describe the functions of each part of our gut in this chapter and include essential accessory organs such as the pancreas, gall bladder and liver, which play a vital role in the absorption and digestion of our food.

The mouth

Food enters our digestive tract through the mouth. In adults the mouth contains 32 teeth whose job it is to tear off food and grind it into smaller pieces. The tongue is a muscular organ used to move food around in the mouth and which has taste buds on its surface to recognize specific tastes. There are also three pairs of salivary glands in the mouth: two **parotid**, two **submandibular** and two **sublingual**. As soon as food enters the mouth, these glands produce saliva, which starts to break down starch. It surprises most people to learn that we produce on average around two litres of saliva every day. It not only breaks down food, it also helps lubricate food and makes it easier to swallow. At the back of the mouth is the **pharynx**: the connection between the mouth and the oesophagus.

The oesophagus

The oesophagus is a muscular tube about 25 centimetres long and 3 centimetres in diameter. It connects the pharynx to the stomach. Food is propelled along its length by muscular contractions known as **peristalsis**. At the lower end of the oesophagus is a strong muscular ring known as the **oesophageal sphincter**, which prevents food from coming back up after it has entered the stomach. It is also designed to keep the stomach acid in the stomach and not refluxing back into the oesophagus.

The stomach

The stomach is a muscular sack about the size of your two fists clenched together. It sits just under the diaphragm (the muscular band which separates your abdomen from your chest cavity) on the left side of your abdomen. The stomach produces hydrochloric acid and digestive enzymes that continue the process of digesting food and breaking it down. Stomach acid is the same pH as battery acid so the stomach produces a thick mucus layer to protect itself from eroding itself. Ridges of muscle called **rugae** line the stomach and when these contract they help to mix up the food.

The small intestine

The small intestine is another muscular tube about 6 metres long and 3 centimetres in diameter. It has three parts: the **duodenum**, the **jejunum** and the **ileum**. The small intestine coils round like a hose and the inner lining is covered in ridges, which increases the surface area and allows maximum absorption. It takes about 6 to 8 hours for food to pass through the stomach and small intestine and during this time about 90 per cent of all the nutrients in our food have been absorbed. The appendix sits at the junction of the end of the small intestine and start of the large intestine. It is between 5 and 10 centimetres long. We don't really know its function, but one theory is that it acts as a sort of reservoir of good bacteria, which can be released after a diarrhoeal illness to reboot our system.

The large intestine

The large intestine is around 1.5 metres long and 8 centimetres in diameter and wraps around the loops of small intestine. Its primary function is to absorb water. Our large bowel also contains 2 kilos of good bacteria called the **gut flora**. These bacteria help to extract the last of the nutrients from our food. It is also in three parts: the **caecum**, the **colon** (ascending, transverse and descending) and the **rectum**. The time it takes for what is left of our food to travel through the intestine is hugely variable and tends to be longer in women than in men. In women it takes an average of 47 hours compared to 33 hours in men and, of course, what you eat can affect that too. Most people will have experienced fast transit times after a very spicy meal, for example.

The liver and gall bladder

The liver is a triangular-shaped organ that sits below the diaphragm on the right side of your abdomen behind the lower ribs. It weighs around 1.5 kilos in healthy adults. One of its many functions is to secrete bile, which is a mixture of water, bile salts, cholesterol and the pigment bilirubin, into the small intestine to aid digestion. There are four lobes in the liver, the left, the right, the caudate and the quadrate lobes, which house 100,000 lobules. Blood enters the liver from the gut through the hepatic portal vein. This blood is rich in sugar, which has been absorbed from our food. The liver absorbs this sugar and stores it in the form of **glycogen**, which can then be used at a later date if sugar levels are low.

The gall bladder is a small pear-shaped organ, which sits below the right lobe of the liver. It is about 8 centimetres long and 1.5 centimetres in diameter. The gall bladder stores and recycles excess bile from the small intestine.

The pancreas

The pancreas sits just below and behind the stomach. It is about 15 centimetres long and it secretes enzymes and hormones to aid digestion and metabolism. About 90 per cent of pancreatic function is to produce digestive enzymes from the **acinar cells**. These enzymes include **proteases** to help digest protein, **lipases** to help digest fat, and **amylases** to help digest carbohydrates. The pancreas also produces hormones from a million islets known as the **islets of Langerhans**. The hormones include **insulin** and **glucagon** to help regulate sugar levels; **somatostatin**, which helps regulate other hormones; and **gastrin**, which helps digestion in the stomach.

What is a normal bowel movement?

There is huge variation between individuals but it is generally accepted that a normal bowel movement is anything between twice a week to three times a day (see Figure 1). The important thing is that you should never need to strain to open your bowels and the stool should be soft. There should never be blood either mixed in with the stool or separately in the pan. If blood is present, you should always get this checked by a doctor. Most cases will be nothing serious but blood in the stool can be a sign of cancer so mustn't be ignored.

Type 1		Separate hard lumps, like nuts (hard to pass)
Type 2		Sausage-shaped but lumpy
Type 3		Like a sausage but with cracks on the surface
Type 4		Like a sausage or snake, smooth and soft
Type 5		Soft blobs with clear-cut edges
Type 6		Fluffy pieces with ragged edges, a mushy stool
Type 7		Watery, no solid pieces. Entirely liquid

Figure 1 Bristol stool chart

Why do I often need to open my bowels after a meal?

A lot of people feel the urge to open their bowels first thing in the morning after breakfast. This is because of a reflex referred to as the **gastrocolic reflex**. As soon as food enters the stomach, stretch receptors are triggered that, in turn, send messages for the muscular gut wall to contract in waves, which propels food through to the intestine. When it reaches the rectum, stretch fibres here recognize that the rectum is now full and this triggers the urge to defecate.

Why does my stomach rumble when I am hungry?

Several hours after a meal when the stomach is empty of food, reflexes trigger a strong wave of muscular contractions. These waves are sometimes referred to as housekeeping movements. They can take over an hour to work their way through the gut and as they do they push fluid and air along the intestine, which can be heard as gurgling sounds.

Why do I feel sleepy after a big meal?

After eating a big meal, especially one that is rich in carbohydrate, a series of messages are sent to the brain triggering the release of serotonin. **Serotonin**, the so called 'happy hormone' makes us feel relaxed and contented.

2

The gastrointestinal system

Examination

What I will describe below is the way we are taught to examine the abdomen at medical school. In truth it is rarely performed this way. In a clinical setting doctors are likely to 'cherry pick' the parts of the examination they think are most likely to help them make a diagnosis. I was once told by a very wise professor that a good doctor gleans most of the important information from talking to the patient. We call this 'taking a history'. If the doctor listens carefully, he or she can fine tune the examination of the patient to the relevant bits and, by the time he or she is ordering tests, a good doctor should have a pretty clear idea of what he or she is looking for. It's an interesting concept and one that I have learned, over the years, to believe in wholeheartedly. It is something worth remembering if you need to see a doctor about gastrointestinal symptoms as these can be the most difficult to differentiate, particularly in the early stages of disease. Spend some time thinking about when your symptoms began, and what makes them worse or better? Note down the treatments you may already have tried and anything else that may be relevant – other medications that you are taking, foreign travel, or friends and family who may have had a similar problem? If you are in pain, is it constant, or does it come and go, and if it does, what seems to trigger it? Is the pain in one spot or does it move anywhere else? And what is the nature of the pain? Is it stabbing or burning? Does it come in spasms or is it like a constant toothache? The more information you can give your doctor about any symptom the better he or she is placed to make a swift diagnosis and get you on the correct treatment as quickly as possible.

Inspection, palpation, percussion and auscultation

Before your doctor touches you, he or she will be looking at you in general. In medical school we were taught that in order to examine the abdomen correctly, it should be exposed 'from nipples to knees'. In General Practice this is rarely necessary and your doctor will want to make you feel at ease so may ask you to expose different areas at different times. You should be lying fairly flat with your arms rested beside you and your doctor will have the examination couch set up so that he or she can examine you from your right hand side. It is amazing what creatures of habit we doctors are. If I do a house call and have to examine a patient from the left side, it feels really wrong! After looking, your doctor will feel, and then he or she may tap his fingers on your abdomen listening to how resonant the sound is (percussion) before listening to your bowel sounds with an stethoscope (auscultation).

The hands

Your doctor will probably start by looking at your hands and you would be surprised what your hands and nails can reveal about your gastrointestinal health. He or she may gently pinch the skin on the back of your hand to assess your state of hydration. Laxity of our skin of course varies with age but if the skin remains raised and doesn't relax quickly this could suggest dehydration. He or she may ask you to place your thumbnails together back to back. There should be a diamond-shaped space between them where the base of the nail passes under the nail fold of skin. If this diamond space is lost, this is called **clubbing**. It can be completely normal but if it develops later in life it can be linked to several diseases in the gastrointestinal system, including Crohn's disease and ulcerative colitis (see Chapter 7) or coeliac disease (see Chapter 6). He or she will also look at your nails. If they are spoon shaped this is called **koilonychias** and can suggest a deficiency of iron. Your doctor will look at the palms of your hands; if they are red this could be linked to liver disease, although there are other common things that will do this too including being pregnant or taking the combined contraceptive pill. He or she will feel in your palm, looking for a band of fibrous tissue in the palm on the side of your little finger. This is called a **Dupuytren's contracture**. It can be something that runs in families, it can be as a result of working with vibrating machinery, but it can also be caused by problems with your liver. He or she may ask you to hold your arms out straight. If your hands start to flap, this is called **asterixis** and is possibly due to liver disease.

The face

Your doctor will look at the whites of the eyes. If there is a yellow tinge, this could be jaundice. He or she may pull down your inner eyelid to look at the colour inside. It should be nice and pink. If it is pale, this could mean anaemia. Yellow plaques around the eyes called **xanthelasma** could mean your cholesterol is raised. If there is a brown-coloured ring around the coloured part of your eye, this is called a **Kayser-Fleischer** ring and can suggest you have a problem with metabolism of copper. If the angles of your mouth are split, this is called **stomatitis** and can mean iron deficiency, which can also cause a sore red tongue referred to as **glossitis**. Your tongue is also a good indicator of your state of hydration. Your doctor may also take note of the smell of your breath. He or she will be checking whether there is a smell of alcohol or a smell like pear drop sweets, which could suggest **ketosis**. This may be as a result of a heavy night on the booze the night before, or can occur in diabetes.

The neck and chest

Your doctor may feel the glands in your neck. One particular gland in the triangle above your collarbone is called **Virchow's node**. If this is swollen it can mean there is an underlying cancer in the abdomen. Your doctor will also look at your skin for evidence of broken blood vessels called **spider naevi**, which can be a sign of liver disease.

The abdomen

So we finally get to the abdomen! Even now your doctor will look first for signs of distension, visible bowel contractions called **peristalsis**, bruises and scars. When your doctor first touches your abdomen he or she will be looking to see if you involuntarily tense your abdominal muscles. This is called **guarding** and suggests what we call an **acute abdomen**, which may require surgery. Your doctor will feel generally; first, making his or her way around your abdomen feeling for areas of tenderness or the presences of any masses. If you are very tender in one area, your doctor may press down on the other side of your abdomen and release the hand quickly. If this causes pain in the original site, this is called **rebound** and is a sign used to check for appendicitis (see Chapter 7). Once your doctor has made a general assessment of your abdomen he or she will check the organs specifically.

- *The liver* Your doctor will use the flat of the hand to feel from the lower right side of your tummy up to the rib cage. A normal healthy liver should sit behind the rib cage or just be felt below it in deep inspiration. Your doctor will ask you to take deep breaths in as he or she feels for an enlarged liver.
- *The gall bladder* If you are very tender in the middle of the lower edge of the liver, this is called a **positive Murphy's sign** which often occurs in the presence of inflammation of the gall bladder, most commonly due to gallstones.

- *The spleen* The spleen lies on the left hand side under the rib cage and examination of it is similar to that for the liver, but on the other side. Your doctor will use the flat of the hand with the fingertips pointing towards the rib cage and move the hand upward asking you to take deep breaths in. If there is any suggestion that the spleen is enlarged, he or she may ask you to roll towards him or her and feel again.
- *The kidneys* The kidneys are examined using two hands. Your doctor will place one hand behind you in the small of your back, and the other on the front of your abdomen trying to feel the kidney between the two hands. This is called **balloting** and unless you are very thin a normal healthy kidney should not be able to be felt in this way.
- *Hernias* Your doctor may ask you to cough while he or she places a hand in your groin to check for hernias.

Once your doctor has finished feeling your abdomen, he or she may place a finger of his or her left hand on your abdomen and tap it with fingers of the other hand. Your doctor is checking for difference in the resonant sound. So if, for example, your doctor suspects an enlarged liver after palpation, he or she may check for a change in sound working his or her way up the abdomen on the right side. Our bowels are full of gas and therefore the sound is resonant compared to a dull sound over solid tissue such as the liver.

The same is true of fluid. In some conditions fluid accumulates in the abdominal cavity. If your doctor suspects this, he or she will use percussion moving from one side of the abdomen to the other. If the sound becomes dull to the sides, your doctor will mark the area and ask you to roll towards him or her while he or she repeats the process. If there is fluid in the cavity, the line where the sound becomes dull will have changed as the fluid has moved with gravity. If he or she suspects **ascites** (accumulation of fluid in the abdominal cavity) your doctor may also try to elicit what is called a **thrill**. Your doctor will place one hand in your flank and then flick the skin on the other side looking for a sensation of an impulse, suggesting underlying fluid which has moved.

Your doctor may then use a stethoscope to listen to your bowel sounds. Normal bowel sounds can be heard gurgling every few seconds but they may be increased in a diarrhoeal illness, or absent in peritonitis. If there is bowel obstruction, a classic tinkling sound may be heard.

The rectum

We were always taught at medical school that no examination of the abdomen was complete without a digital examination of the rectum. In fact, they used to say 'if you don't put your finger in it, you could put your foot in it'. That sounds horribly flippant but what our tutors meant was that it is easy to miss a rectal cancer if you don't specifically check for it. We certainly don't examine the rectum in every patient with gastrointestinal symptoms in General Practice. It isn't necessary if the diagnosis is clear. But if there is any chance your symptoms could be linked to a cancer your doctor will have to feel inside your rectum with a finger. It may not be the most pleasant thing, but it could save your life.

Tests

After your doctor has taken a full history of your symptoms and concerns and examined you, he or she may want to do some tests. Some of these tests, such as blood tests and certain X-rays and scans, can be arranged by your GP. Others will need a referral to a specialist. Your doctor will explain what will happen and should be able to give you an idea of time frame. It is important that you make sure that you know the plan. For example, is it up to you to make a follow up appointment with your GP after you have had the tests? If this is the case, you also need to know how long it is likely to be before your GP will receive the results. There is nothing more frustrating for all concerned than if you make an appointment to receive your results and they have not yet been sent to your surgery.

Below is a list of the sort of tests you may go through.

Blood tests

There are several blood tests that can be done to check the health of your gastrointestinal system. This doesn't mean several needles though. Your doctor may do some blood tests there and then, but he or she is more likely to ask you to re-book with the practice nurse, who will take the blood samples needed. She will place a tourniquet around your upper arm and tighten it to occlude the veins and make them swell so that they are easier to see. She may ask you to open and close your fist, which also helps dilate the veins. She will then use an alcohol wipe to clean the skin. The most common place used to take blood is the inside of the elbow. This is called the **antecubital fossa**. She will use a sterile needle to puncture the vein and collect blood samples into different bottles depending which tests are being done. This shouldn't be painful but in young children I often use an anaesthetic cream on the skin for 20 to 30 minutes before the test to numb the skin. If your doctor suggests this, it is worth putting the cream on the inner aspects of both elbows and on the backs of both hands so that there are plenty of options if the veins are difficult to see.

Stool samples

There are two main reasons we arrange stool samples. One is to check for infection. Your doctor will ask you to collect a sample of faeces into a small tube for analysis under a microscope, looking for microorganisms that cause food poisoning and gastroenteritis. The sample is also cultured in a laboratory to see if bugs can be grown so it can take some time for the results to come back.

The other reason is to look for microscopic traces of blood in the stool. In this instance, you will be given three stool sample pots and be asked to collect samples from your faeces on three separate occasions and preferably from different areas of the stool. These are then sent to the lab to look for traces of blood. If blood is present, there could be a polyp or even a cancer in the gastrointestinal tract so your doctor will want to arrange further tests to look into this.

If you are registered with an NHS GP and aged between 60 and 69 you will be sent a simple stool sample kit as a routine screening test every two years. Sadly, only about half of all the kits that are sent out are returned. I guess that's because the idea of collecting your poo and smearing it on a card is not most people's idea of fun. It may not be but – honestly – it is a test that could save your life. Bowel cancer is totally curable if caught early, so, please, when your time comes, take the test.

Proctoscopy

Some would argue that a proctoscopy is part of a complete abdominal examination and it is certainly something that can be done in the GP surgery. A small instrument that looks like a clear plastic tube is inserted into the anus. You will be asked to strain down and your doctor will look for dilated purple veins, which could be **haemorrhoids**, splits in the skin called **fissures**, or tumours.

Sigmoidoscopy

A sigmoidoscopy involves inserting a longer instrument into the anus. This is either a rigid tube about 25 centimetres long (called a **rigid sigmoidoscopy**) or a flexible tube about 60 centimetres long (a **flexible sigmoidoscopy**). The rigid sigmoidoscopy can be performed without what we call bowel preparation but the flexible sigmoidoscopy requires the patient to take laxatives before the procedure to clear out the bowel and allow for a better view. Once the instrument is inserted into the anus, rectum and beyond, air is pumped into the sigmoid colon and the doctor can see the lining of this part of the colon under direct vision. In patients suffering with irritable bowel syndrome, the passing of this air can reproduce the pain that they experience and while this is not a diagnostic test, it can be an indicator of this diagnosis.

Colonoscopy

This is a more invasive procedure, which requires more preparation. You will be asked to drink only fluids for 24 hours before a colonoscopy and your doctor will give you sachets of a strong laxative to take to ensure that the bowel is empty. You will be given a sedative to have the procedure, which will take 15 to 30 minutes, during which the doctor will hope to examine your colon all the way up to your caecum or ileum. If you are due to have this procedure make sure that you arrange to be taken and collected from the hospital as you will be unable to drive after the sedation.

Gastroscopy

A gastroscopy is done to examine your stomach under direct vision using a special telescope. You should stop any medicines prescribed for indigestion at least two weeks before. You will be asked to fast for 4 hours prior to the procedure to ensure that you stomach is empty. The doctor will spray an anaesthetic spray into the back of your throat to numb your gag reflex and he or she will then pass the gastroscope over the back of your tongue and down your oesophagus into your stomach. Most people choose to have this done under local sedation. This simply involves an injection into the back of your hand but, just as with a colonoscopy, it will mean that you won't be allowed to go home alone so you will need to find someone to accompany you.

X-rays

Abdominal X-rays are particularly useful if we suspect an acute abdomen. This occurs in peritonitis or bowel perforation, where we can see characteristic patterns of gas collection. Constipation can also be seen on a plain abdominal X-ray, as can gallstones, although a computerized tomography (CT) scan is more accurate for the latter.

Ultrasound scans

Ultrasound scans are very good at detecting fluid collections. They can also pick up dilated loops of bowel, which are seen when the bowel is obstructed. They are also used to guide your doctor if he or she is trying to biopsy a particular area. An ultrasound involves lying on your back on an examination couch. The radiographer will put some special clear jelly on your tummy to allow better transmission of the ultrasound waves and will use a probe over the skin of your abdomen which relays pictures back to a screen. Ultrasound probes can also be incorporated into gastroscopes or endoscopes to examine the oesophagus or rectum, respectively.

CT scans

CT scans involve significantly more radiation than ultrasound scans. You will be asked to lie on your back as a tube rotates around you. You may also be asked to move positions so that the radiographer can get different views. The whole thing should only take about 10 minutes, and, as it doesn't involve lying in a tunnel, most people find no problem with it. CT scans are very good at detecting small collections of fluid or gas and at looking at the bowel wall. They are sometimes used with an injection of contrast dye. They are often used to confirm an appendicitis, diverticulitis or Crohn's disease and are very useful in staging cancers so that we know just how far the cancer has spread before deciding on the most appropriate treatment.

MRI scans

MRI stands for **magnetic resonance imaging** and involves no radiation, but it does involve lying in a long tube, which some people find claustrophobic. It can take anything from 15 to 90 minutes and you will need to stay as still as possible as any movement will distort the images. You will be able to speak to the radiographer throughout the procedure through an intercom. Some centres now have open MRI scanners, which are open on three sides so are less claustrophobic. MRIs are particularly useful for examining the small bowel, liver and gall bladder, and rectum.

PET scans

A PET (**positron emission tomography**) scan involves either an injection of, or breathing in, a radioactive substance known as a **radiotracer**. This will take 30 to 90 minutes to work its way around your body. After this, you will be asked to lie on a bed, which is then moved through a circular scanner. This should take 30 to 60 minutes, during which time you should lie as still as possible and not talk. The amount of radiation used is completely safe and you shouldn't experience any side effects. PET scans are generally used to stage oesophageal, gastric or rectal cancers.

Barium studies

Barium studies involve either drinking a substance that glows white on X-ray or having the substance as an enema. Ulcers show up as a pooling of the white fluid. If a tumour or a structure is present, this may show as a narrowing of the white fluid.

3

The mouth

Ulcers

Mouth ulcers are extremely common, particularly in women and young adults, and most people will experience them at some point in their lives. They usually form on the inside of the lips or the cheeks and are oval shaped. They can be red, white or grey in the middle, and are sore especially when you eat or drink.

What causes mouth ulcers?

There is often no specific cause identified. Sometimes they can be due to trauma in the mouth when you inadvertently bite your lip or cheek, or burn yourself with hot food or drinks. Sometimes they can be caused by poorly fitting dentures. They also seem to be linked to stress in some people and for some women they occur around the time of your period. In susceptible people, certain foods can trigger them, including caffeine, nuts, cheese, strawberries, tomatoes, chocolate and wheat flour. Some people find mouth ulcers flare up when they first stop smoking, but don't let this put you off if you are trying to give up smoking – this is short lived. Occasionally there is a specific cause such as a deficiency in iron, Crohn's disease (see Chapter 7) or coeliac disease (see Chapter 6). They can also be caused by some medicines, infection and, rarely, they are cancerous.

What can I do to prevent mouth ulcers?

Try keeping a diary to see if you can identify what causes mouth ulcers for you. If you identify certain foods then try cutting them out for a while. Learning to manage your stress is also important, as is eating a well balanced diet including iron-rich foods such as red meat and green leafy vegetables.

How can I treat mouth ulcers?

Most mouth ulcers will heal of their own accord in two weeks but they can be very sore during this time so you may want to invest in a softer toothbrush. Avoid spicy or acidic foods as these are likely to cause pain. Interestingly liquorice has natural ulcer-healing properties so if you like liquorice now is the perfect excuse to indulge! Your pharmacist can also advise about topical gels to help, and antiseptic mouth-washes to prevent any secondary infection in the ulcer.

When should I see my doctor?

If the simple measures above are not helping then your doctor can prescribe steroid lozenges to reduce the inflammation. The vast majority of ulcers are nothing to worry about but an ulcer that persists for more than three weeks should always be checked by your doctor or dentist as oral cancer can present as a persistent mouth ulcer.

Salivary stones

There are three pairs of salivary glands in the mouth – the parotid, the submandibular and the sublingual. Over three-quarters of salivary stones occur in the submandibular glands. Most are very small (less than 1 millimetre) but they can cause significant pain. We don't know why they form but they can cause blockage of the salivary duct, which means that every time you eat and produce saliva there is a back pressure because the saliva cannot get past the blockage into the mouth. The stones are made of calcium but they are not linked to high calcium levels in the diet or in the blood. Because they are made of calcium, they show up white on plain X-rays but one in five stones doesn't show on a plain film. If your doctor still suspects a stone he or she may arrange something called a **sialogram**. This is where a tiny plastic tube is inserted from the mouth into the salivary duct. A dye that shows up on X-ray is then injected into the gland. The tube is then removed and X-rays are taken to look for a blockage.

Can salivary stones be treated?

Sometimes small stones pass into the mouth without the need for treatment. The patient may be aware of a gritty sensation in the mouth but nothing else. If stones don't pass, they can sometimes be dislodged by using a small probe in the salivary duct. More resistant stones may need to be removed with a procedure called a **sialendoscopy**. This involves inserting a tiny telescope into the salivary duct. A grabber can be inserted along the telescope to literally grab the stone and pull it out. Occasionally, if this doesn't work, you will need surgery to remove the stone. In some centres they also use shock wave treatment called **lithotripsy** to break stones down into tiny pieces, which are then easier to pass.

Will the stones recur?

Most salivary stones don't recur but if you are unlucky enough to have a recurrent problem, your specialist might talk to you about an operation to remove the whole gland. You have five others so you will still produce enough saliva, and once you have recovered from the operation, you won't be aware of any difference.

Glossitis

Glossitis simply means inflammation of the tongue. It presents itself as a sore red tongue which may look smoother than normal. Patients often tell me that their food tastes metallic as well. Common causes include deficiencies of vitamin B2, B12 or iron. It can sometimes be caused by infection with a fungus called *Candida albicans*. This is known as **oral thrush** and is most common in diabetics, people taking steroids, people with problems with their immune system, or those who have been on antibiotics.

What should I do if I think I may have glossitis?

It is important that you see your GP if you think you could have glossitis as your doctor may want to do some tests to work out why this has happened. The treatment will depend on the cause and your doctor will advise you on your individual case.

What is black hairy tongue?

Our mouths are full of bacteria, which are kept in balance. In some people the bacteria overgrow and the result is a brown staining of the tongue known as **black hairy tongue.** It is more common in smokers and those who overuse antiseptic mouthwashes. It isn't serious but people find it understandably distressing. Stopping smoking and cutting back on the mouthwashes will help.

What is geographic tongue?

A geographic tongue is where there are areas of the tongue that look more red and appear to have a raised area surrounding them, making the tongue look like a map – hence the name. We don't know why it happens but it occurs in about one in a hundred British adults and may run in families, but there are no serious implications and it is nothing to worry about.

Halitosis

Halitosis is the medical term for bad breath. It is something we will all suffer from at some point, but for some people it is an ongoing problem that can cause a lot of distress.

How do I know if I've got bad breath?

The simplest way to know is to ask someone close to you but if you would rather not, you can use a teaspoon to scrape the back of your tongue and smell it yourself immediately. If there is an unpleasant odour, then you have halitosis.

What causes halitosis?

By far the commonest cause of bad breath is poor dental hygiene and if you are concerned about the smell of your breath, then a visit to your dentist and the hygienist should be your first port of call. It is also common to have bad breath first thing in the morning but if your breath is fresh after cleaning your teeth and flossing, then you have nothing to worry about. Other causes include those listed below.

- *Food and drink* Alcohol, spicy foods, garlic and coffee are the most common culprits here. For most people this is a transient problem and not one that causes much concern but if you consume a lot of these the problem may become more of an issue.
- *Smoking* Ask anyone who lives with a smoker, or even better an ex-smoker, and they will tell you what they think of the smell of stale smoke on a person's breath!
- *Medicines* Some medicines, particularly those that give you a dry mouth, can predispose to bad breath.
- *Fasting* If you go without food for a prolonged period, your body will use up fat stores for energy and the by-products of this are **ketones**. Ketones have a characteristic smell similar to pear drop sweets and can be smelled on your breath.

- *Infections* Tonsillitis is the most common one here, but infection anywhere in the oral cavity or the lungs can cause bad breath.
- *Fish odour syndrome* This is a rare condition where the body has a faulty gene and cannot break down a substance called **trimethylamine**, which is found in foods such as eggs, seafood, liver, kidney, peas, beans, sprouts, broccoli, cauliflower and cabbage, peanuts and soy products.

Anyone with bad breath needs to take a visit to the dentist before anything else. After that it is about working out the cause and acting accordingly but if you think your prescription medicine may be to blame, please don't just stop it. Make an appointment to see your GP to discuss alternatives.

Mouth cancer

Cancer can occur anywhere in the mouth – lips, cheeks, tongue or gums. It usually occurs in people over 50 and is more common in men than women. It may start as a lump, an ulcer or just an area of red or white. These symptoms are relatively common and in the vast majority of cases are caused by something other than cancer, but if you notice something like this in your mouth which doesn't resolve within three weeks then you should always get it checked out by your GP or dentist.

What causes mouth cancer?

Your risks of developing mouth cancer increase if you:

- smoke or chew tobacco products;
- drink alcohol to excess;
- chew betel nut;
- have been infected with the human papilloma virus (HPV);
- have poor oral hygiene;
- have a poor diet.

How is mouth cancer diagnosed?

If your doctor or dentist suspects mouth cancer they will arrange for a biopsy (a sample of tissue) to be taken, under local anaesthetic, and be sent for examination under a microscope in the laboratory.

How is mouth cancer treated?

There are various treatments available and most patients will have a combination of two or more of them. If caught early sometimes the cancer can be treated with laser therapy. Surgery is sometimes used to remove the tumour and some of the surrounding healthy tissue. Many mouth cancers are sensitive to radiotherapy and this may be used either alone or after surgery. Mouth cancer usually requires daily treatments for anything up to seven weeks and can leave your mouth feeling sore and dry, but this usually passes when you have finished the course. If your cancer has spread or your doctors are concerned there is a high risk of the cancer recurring, you may also be offered chemotherapy.

4

The oesophagus

Indigestion

Indigestion (or to use its medical term, **dyspepsia**) is one of the most common gastroenterological complaints. It usually presents as a burning sensation in the upper abdomen, which may radiate through to the back. It may also cause a feeling of nausea and the need to belch. Most of us will experience indigestion at some point, but for some people it is a daily problem which interferes with their quality of life.

What causes indigestion?

There are lots of causes of dyspepsia. Being overweight, smoking, drinking alcohol to excess, and a diet rich in very spicy foods are likely to exacerbate symptoms. There are a number of underlying conditions that can cause dyspepsia. I will discuss them in greater depth in this chapter and the next but they include:

- acid reflux, often referred to as GORD (gastro-oesophageal reflux disease);
- oesophagitis, inflammation of the oesophagus;
- gastritis, inflammation of the stomach;
- duodenitis, inflammation of the duodenum – the first part of the small intestine;
- hiatus hernia (see Chapter 5);
- infection with *H. pylori* (see Chapter 5);
- medication, non-steroidal anti-inflammatory drugs and steroids are some of the most common culprits here;
- peptic ulcers, ulcers in the stomach or duodenum;
- Barrett's oesophagus;
- stomach and oesophageal cancer.

Who gets indigestion?

Anyone can get indigestion. It is more common if you are overweight, if you smoke, and if you drink alcohol above the recommended limits, which are just 14 units a week for women and 21 units a week for men. That is probably less than you think. To calculate the number of units you are drinking, you simply need to look at the percentage alcohol of the drink you are drinking. That equates to the number of units in a litre of that fluid. So, to make the maths easy, let's say you are drinking 12 per cent wine. That means there are 12 units in a litre and therefore 9 units in a standard 75 cl (3/4 of a litre) bottle. If you were to pour yourself a glass of wine at home, it is likely to be a large (250 millilitres) one. That is one-third of a bottle, namely one-third of 9, which is 3 units, not the single unit that you probably previously thought it was. And, of course, if you do that every day that is your total allowance, if you are a man and 50 per cent more than the recommended limits if you are a woman!

How can I treat indigestion?

There are some simple things that you can do for yourself to alleviate your symptoms. Cut back on alcohol and stop smoking if you can. Try to maintain a healthy body mass index (BMI). Manage your stress, as stress will increase stomach acid production. Try propping up the head of your bed on blocks so that gravity is working in your favour when you go to bed. Avoid eating large meals late at night, and speak to your pharmacist about products available over the counter to combat acid.

When should I see my doctor?

Indigestion is very common and most cases can be managed between you and your pharmacist, but you should see your doctor if:

- you vomit blood;

- you are losing weight unintentionally;
- your stools look black and tarry (this could mean old blood in the stool);
- you are over 55 and have persistent or unexplained indigestion;
- you have difficulty swallowing;
- you feel generally unwell and exhausted.

Gastro-oesophageal reflux disease (GORD)

Gastro-oesophageal reflux disease (which I will refer to as GORD from now on) is a common condition where acid refluxes from the stomach into the oesophagus, which is not designed to withstand such strong acid, and this therefore causes symptoms. The classic symptoms include a burning pain in the top of the abdomen, known medically as the **epigastrium**, an unpleasant acidic taste in the mouth and pain on swallowing, especially hot and spicy foods. Occasionally it presents as a persistent cough, which is generally worse at night when lying down. I have lost count of the people I have treated with antacid medication for a persistent cough. They usually look at me as though I have finally lost my marbles but, more often than not, are pleasantly surprised when the cough disappears.

Why does GORD happen?

It is usually caused by a weakness in the muscular sphincter at the bottom of the oesophagus. If this is working well it prevents the strong stomach acid from burning the lining of the oesophagus, but if it is weakened then acid can reflux back and this is most common in people who are overweight, eating a high fat diet, or pregnant.

How is GORD diagnosed?

In most cases GORD can be diagnosed on the history alone so take some time thinking about your symptoms before your appointment. If you can describe accurately where you feel the pain, what type of pain it is and what makes it worse or better, your GP will be more easily able to distinguish between the possible explanations. Having made the diagnosis, your doctor will probably be able to give you a trial of treatment straight away and the most commonly used drugs are called **proton pump inhibitors** (PPIs). There are several different PPIs and they are designed to switch off the acid in your stomach and therefore allow any inflammation to heal. They are very effective and in my experience people often feel so much better within a few days that they forget to continue. I always stress that it is important to complete the course as you need to allow time for the inflammation to settle otherwise even a small amount of acid can bring back symptoms with a vengeance.

Will I need an endoscopy?

Most people with GORD will not need an endoscopy but if you have what doctors refer to as 'red flag' signs, you will be referred for an endoscopy to make sure there isn't anything more serious going on. Red flag symptoms include:

- unexplained weight loss
- gastrointestinal bleeding
- unexplained anaemia
- persistent vomiting
- difficulty swallowing
- a lump in the abdomen.

If you are booked for an endoscopy, your doctor will probably ask you to stop your medication for a couple of weeks before the procedure.

Mallory Weiss tear

Unless you or someone you know has had a Mallory Weiss tear it is probably not a condition you will have heard of, but it is a condition that occurs in people who are repeatedly sick or who cough. In fact, anything that persistently raises the pressure in the stomach or lower oesophagus can lead to a tear in the delicate lining of the upper gastrointestinal tract. It has also been seen in people with epilepsy, for example.

What are the symptoms of a Malory Weiss?

The most common presentation is for an individual to vomit fresh red blood, which is understandably very frightening at the time. This usually occurs after a bout of repeated retching or vomiting. It can also be followed by the passage of tarry-looking black stools where some blood is swallowed and takes on the dark appearance of altered blood as it makes its way through the gut.

How is a Mallory Weiss diagnosed?

Your doctor will probably arrange for an endoscopy if he or she suspects a tear. If one is present it can be viewed under direct vision through the endoscope and the doctor can see if the bleeding has settled or not. If there is no further bleeding, you will probably just be kept in hospital for a while to ensure everything has settled but shouldn't need any further intervention. If, however, the bleeding persists, you may need a small operation to seal off the bleeding. This can be done with clips, bands, lasers, injections or a heated probe. Exactly which procedure will be decided upon by your specialist. The good news is that once healed it is unusual for a Mallory Weiss to recur.

Achalasia

Food gets from the mouth to the anus by muscular contractions in the gut wall known as **peristalsis**. Achalasia is a condition where those contractions in the wall of the oesophagus don't work properly. In addition, the muscular sphincter between the bottom of the oesophagus and the stomach doesn't open properly and as a result food gets stuck in the oesophagus. We don't really know why it happens but it seems to be due to damage to the nerves supplying the muscles. One theory is that this could be caused by a viral infection. Another is that it may be linked to problems with the immune system.

What are the symptoms of achalasia?

The symptoms depend on the severity of the condition. In the early stages, you may not be aware of a problem but as things progress you are likely to notice that food appears to get stuck in your gullet. You may regurgitate food and as it progresses you may lose weight as you are unable to digest your food properly.

How is achalasia diagnosed?

If your doctor suspects achalasia, he or she will probably arrange for you to have a barium swallow. This involves drinking some barium, which shows up white on an X-ray. You will then have a series of X-rays taken to show the passage of the barium as it passes through your upper gastro-intestinal tract. The radiologists will be looking for a delay in the passage of barium from your oesophagus into the stomach. You may also be offered an endoscopy. During this procedure, the doctor will be looking for trapped food lodged at the base of the oesophagus. We can also use a special technique called **manometry** to measure the pressure in the oesophagus and at the sphincter.

How is achalasia treated?

Once the diagnosis is confirmed, your doctor will talk through the treatment options with you. Some people respond to tablets to relax the sphincter of muscle at the base of the oesophagus, but others may need a small operation to stretch the sphincter under general anaesthetic. This is usually successful but may need repeating. Alternatively, some specialists use injections of botulinum toxin to relax the muscle. This works but needs repeating at regular intervals. Occasionally a keyhole operation is required to physically divide the muscle fibres.

Is there anything I can do to help myself?

If you have achalasia or are recovering from a treatment for the condition, it is important that you take time to eat your meals and chew your food properly. Make sure you take plenty of fluids with every meal. At night try to sleep propped up on pillows or raise the head of your bed on blocks so that you have gravity on your side.

Are there any long-term problems with achalasia?

If achalasia is ignored and food is wedged in the gullet, it can be regurgitated at night and if, then, it inadvertently goes back into the lungs, it can cause choking or a chest infection. Long term, if the symptoms of achalasia are ignored and food is allowed to accumulate in the oesophagus, then there is an increased risk of developing cancer of the oesophagus so it is important not to ignore these symptoms and get them sorted out.

Oesophageal webs, rings and strictures

All of these conditions can cause narrowing of the oesophagus. Oesophageal webs are abnormalities of the lining of the oesophagus, rings are abnormalities of the muscular layer and strictures are caused by scarring, usually from acid reflux, and can be benign or cancerous (malignant). The narrowing can cause difficulty swallowing (dysphagia) and this must always be investigated because of the possibility of cancer. A combination of barium studies and endoscopy confirms the presence of an obstruction and if there is any possibility of cancer, a biopsy can be taken at the time of endoscopy. Benign strictures can also be treated with dilation at the time of endoscopy while cancer needs more aggressive treatment (see below).

Barrett's oesophagus

Barrett's oesophagus is a term used to describe a change in the cells lining the oesophagus, which is caused by acid refluxing into the oesophagus. It is important because it is associated with a risk that some of those cells could become cancerous, so it is important that the diagnosis is recognized and individuals are monitored. The risk is low – less than 5 per cent of people with Barrett's will go on to develop cancer but of course, if that is you, it is a huge deal, so it is better to be safe than sorry. In the past we monitored patients with regular endoscopy but now we have a technique called the **cytosponge**, which is much simpler and less invasive for patients. You simply swallow a capsule containing a sponge, which is left in place for 5 minutes. During this time the outer capsule dissolves and then the sponge is pulled back up on a thread. As the sponge is retrieved it collects cells from the lining of the oesophagus, which can then be analysed in the laboratory for signs of Barrett's.

Who gets Barrett's oesophagus?

Anyone who has problems with reflux could be at risk, so people who are overweight, smokers, people who drink alcohol excessively and those that eat large amounts of very spicy or fatty foods are all at risk.

How would I know if I had Barrett's?

You may not is the simple answer, which is why it is so important that you don't ignore long-term symptoms of indigestion.

What is the treatment for Barrett's?

Your doctor will want to make sure you do all you can to reduce your acid reflux so will talk to you about weight management, healthy eating, giving up smoking and cutting back on alcohol. He may also prescribe medication to reduce your acid production. You will also need to have the abnormal cells removed. This can be done via an endoscope using a thin wire called a snare, radio waves, heat treatment or light therapy.

Oesophageal cancer

There are two types of oesophageal cancer, both of which are, thankfully, not common but they are becoming significantly more frequent here in the UK so it is important that we cover them in this chapter. The most common form starts in the mucous glands lining the oesophagus. This is called **adenocarcinoma**. It tends to form in the lower third of the oesophagus and accounts for 60 per cent of all cases of carcinoma of the oesophagus. The other 40 per cent of cases start in the cells lining the oesophagus and this is called **squamous cell carcinoma**.

Who gets oesophageal cancer?

There is no one specific cause for oesophageal cancer but we do know that there are several factors that increase the risk of it developing. These include:

- age, most cases occur in the over 55 age group;
- gender, it is more common in men than in women;
- geography, oesophageal cancer is more common in China, for example, than it is in the UK although we don't yet know why that should be;
- alcohol, heavy drinkers and especially heavy spirit drinkers are most at risk;
- smoking, the more you smoke the greater the risk;
- Barrett's oesophagus (see above);

- GORD, long-term exposure of the oesophagus to acid increases the risk;
- flushing, people who flush (or blush) when they drink alcohol lack an enzyme called **aldehyde dehydrogenase 2** and one study has drawn a link between this and developing oesophageal cancer.

What are the symptoms of oesophageal cancer?

In the early stages you may not have any symptoms but as the cancer grows you are likely to find a difficulty swallowing food. Initially this will be very solid food but if left untreated this will include softer foods and even, ultimately, liquids. You are likely to lose weight unintentionally. You may be sick frequently and sometimes the vomit may contain blood. Some people develop a cough or a hoarse voice.

How is oesophageal cancer diagnosed?

The initial diagnosis is likely to be made on endoscopy. The doctor will biopsy any suspicious-looking areas so that they can be examined under the microscope. If a cancer is confirmed on biopsy, the specialists will then arrange for various scans and other tests to check how far (if at all) the cancer has spread.

What will the treatment involve?

Your treatment will depend on the extent of the cancer and how far it has spread. Your overall general health will also be taken into consideration and you should be involved in the decision-making along the way. If you are in reasonable physical health and the tumour has been caught early enough, you will be offered surgery to remove the cancer aiming for a cure. Even if the whole cancer cannot be removed your specialist may suggest he or she removes what he or she can to alleviate symptoms, or that he or she puts a rigid tube through the tumour called a **stent**. This will allow food to pass into the stomach. You may also be offered chemotherapy or radiotherapy.

5

The stomach

Hiatus hernia

The oesophagus lies in the chest cavity and the stomach lies in the abdominal cavity. The two are separated by a thick layer of muscle called the **diaphragm** with a small hole in the middle to accommodate the gastro-oesophageal junction. A hiatus hernia is where part of the stomach slides through this hole to sit in the chest cavity. There are two main types:

- *sliding*, this is the most common type accounting for about 90 per cent of all hiatus hernias. This is where the junction between stomach and oesophagus and part of the stomach slide through the diaphragm up into the chest.
- *rolling*, this is where just part of the stomach rolls through hole to lie next to the oesophagus.

A sliding hiatus hernia is likely to cause more problems with symptoms of GORD (Chapter 4) as the delicate oesophageal lining is exposed to stomach acid. A rolling hiatus hernia, however, leaves the muscular sphincter intact.

How is a hiatus hernia diagnosed?

If your doctor suspects a hiatus hernia he or she can confirm this with either an endoscopy or a barium study.

What is the treatment for a hiatus hernia?

There is quite a lot you can do to help yourself. If you are overweight, losing weight to achieve a healthy BMI will take the pressure off your stomach and ease symptoms. Try to avoid eating large meals especially late at night and prop the head of your bed up so that you have gravity on your side. Speak to your pharmacist about antacid medications and if these don't work, your GP can prescribe alternatives. Occasionally, if symptoms are really interfering with your quality of life you may be offered an operation to put the stomach back where it should be and strengthen the gastro-oesophageal sphincter.

Gastritis

Gastritis is inflammation (*itis*) of the stomach (*gastrum*) and it is extremely common. It can occur very suddenly, in which case we call it 'acute', or can be more long standing, which is called 'chronic'. It's interesting that in lay speech both acute and chronic are words that are used to express severity, but in medical terms they are used in term of time frame, with acute always meaning short term and chronic meaning more long term.

What causes gastritis?

There are lots of different causes of gastritis. In most cases there will probably be a combination of factors that trigger an attack and these can include any of:

- alcohol
- stress
- smoking
- cocaine use
- chronic vomiting
- hot spicy foods
- infection
- bile
- pernicious anaemia
- medications, especially non-steroidal anti-inflammatory drugs and steroids.

The most common infection responsible is something called *Helicobacter pylori* (see below).

How would I know if I had gastritis?

The most common symptoms associated with gastritis are indigestion and abdominal pain. There may also be nausea and sometimes vomiting. Patients often tell me they typically wake in the early hours with a burning sensation in the upper abdomen. Many have worked out that if they keep a glass of milk and a biscuit beside the bed to take at times like this the symptoms improve. This is because the milk neutralizes the stomach acid.

How is gastritis treated?

The first thing to do is to look at all the triggers listed above and avoid any that you think may be relevant to you. Don't stop any prescription medication without speaking to your doctor first. It can be dangerous to suddenly stop steroids so make sure you discuss things first. Lots of patients can manage their condition with lifestyle changes and over the counter medicines but if these don't control your symptoms, you will need to see your GP for an alternative prescription.

Do I need to see my doctor?

If your symptoms are controlled with simple measures, there is no need to see your GP, but you must go if:

- your symptoms persist despite taking the measures above;
- you are losing weight unexpectedly;
- you vomit blood;
- your stools go black and tarry (this could be bleeding from within the stomach).

Helicobacter pylori (*H. pylori*)

Helicobacter pylori infection is the most common cause of stomach ulcers. I remember its discovery! A doctor in Australia was so convinced that he had made a medical breakthrough and that he knew the common cause of stomach ulcers that he actually drank a cocktail of this bacteria and induced an ulcer in himself! *H. pylori* is a very common bacterium. About half the world's population has it and once you have contracted it, unless you are treated, you are likely to have it for life.

How would I know if I had *H. pylori*?

The infection itself won't cause any symptoms but about 15 per cent of people infected develop problems with indigestion and may even develop ulcers in the stomach or duodenum. We are not exactly sure how this comes about but one theory is that the bacteria interfere with the mucous lining that protects the stomach. It can also increase the risk of stomach cancer.

How is *H. pylori* diagnosed?

If your doctor suspects *H. pylori* infection, he or she may arrange something called a **urea breath test**. *H. pylori* can break down urea to produce carbon dioxide, which is then eliminated in your breath. You will be asked to swallow a capsule containing urea made from a special form of carbon known as an **isotope**. If *H. pylori* is in your stomach, the urea in the capsule will be broken down. The carbon will be absorbed and will be made into carbon dioxide, which you will exhale. Samples of your exhaled breath will be collected and if the isotope is present in the exhaled carbon dioxide, you have *H. pylori* infection. This test can also be repeated after treatment to confirm that the bacteria has been eradicated. There are also blood tests available looking for antibodies to *H. pylori*.

What happens if I test positive?

If you test positive, you will be offered what we call eradication therapy, which involves taking a course of medication including something called a **proton pump inhibitor**, to

switch off acid production in your stomach, and a combination of antibiotics. You may be asked to repeat the breath test
after completing your treatment to check that the infection
has cleared.

Peptic ulcers

Ulcers in the lower oesophagus, stomach or first part of the
small intestine (the duodenum) are called **peptic ulcers**.

Who gets peptic ulcers?

Anyone can get a peptic ulcer. They are very common. In
fact one in ten UK adults will have an ulcer at some point
in their lives. Most are caused by infection with *H. pylori* (see
above) or from the use of non-steroidal anti-inflammatory
drugs such as aspirin or ibuprofen, which are known to irritate the stomach lining. Stress, alcohol and smoking will also
increase your risk.

How would I know if I had a peptic ulcer?

The most common symptom is a burning pain usually felt
at the top of your stomach and sometimes also felt going
through to your back. It is often worse just after eating when
the stomach produces acid to aid digestion, and can last for
anything from a few minutes to several hours. Patients often
tell me they wake in the early hours with this pain, and
drinking milk or taking an antacid helps alleviate the pain.
You may also feel nauseous and at its worst you may vomit
blood or notice that your stools become black and tarry
looking. This is called **melaena**. The appearance is due to old
blood, which has come from bleeding in the upper gut and
turned black (just like a scab) in the time it has taken to travel
the length of the intestine.

What should I do if I suspect an ulcer?

If your symptoms are mild, you may be able to manage them by speaking to your pharmacist about antacid medication and making some lifestyle changes including giving up smoking, cutting back on alcohol and managing your stress. If, however, your symptoms persist despite these measures, you will need to see your GP. You should also see your doctor if you vomit blood or develop melaena.

What will my doctor do?

If your doctor suspects an ulcer, he or she will probably arrange an endoscopy to look into the upper gut. Your doctor may also test for *H. pylori*. Depending on the result of the tests, he or she will then arrange treatment, which may involve a proton pump inhibitor (PPI) to switch off the acid production in your stomach and allow the ulcer to heal, or *H. pylori* eradication therapy. In the past, a lot of people ended up needing surgery for an ulcer but since the advent of PPIs and our knowledge of *H. pylori*, this is rarely needed today.

Are there any long-term problems with peptic ulcers?

If ignored, there is the possibility that an ulcer could perforate through the lining of the gut and this is a medical emergency. Stomach ulcers can also increase your risk of developing stomach cancer.

Stomach cancer

Stomach cancer is relatively uncommon but, like all cancers, the sooner it is detected, the better the outlook.

Who gets stomach cancer?

There are a number of factors that increase your risk and these include:

- *gender*, men are twice as likely as women to develop stomach cancer;

- *age*, most cases occur in the over 55s;
- *smoking*, people who smoke are twice as likely to develop stomach cancer;
- *H. pylori* infection;
- *stomach ulcers*;
- *family history*, if you have a close relative with stomach cancer, this doubles your risk;
- *diet*, a diet rich in pickled vegetables, salt and smoked meats increases your risk;
- *blood type A*, if you are blood type A this is associated with an increased risk;
- *another cancer*, having another cancer including cancer of the bowel, prostate, bladder, testicle, breast, ovary or cervix can also increase your risk.

How is stomach cancer diagnosed?

Your doctor will arrange an endoscopy and if there is suspicion that there is cancer then biopsies will be taken at the time for analysis in the laboratory. You may also have an ultrasound test and a barium swallow. If these confirm cancer, then your doctors will arrange further tests, which will probably include a CT or MRI scan to assess whether the cancer has spread outside the stomach as this will affect the treatment you will need.

How is stomach cancer treated?

You may need to have all or part of your stomach removed surgically and then you will probably be offered chemotherapy or radiotherapy. A complete cure is achievable in up to a third of cases.

6

The small intestine

Coeliac disease

Coeliac disease is a lifelong condition caused by an immune reaction to gluten, resulting in inflammation of the gut lining. It is often described as an allergy but strictly speaking, it is not an allergy or even an intolerance. It is what we call an autoimmune disease, where the body develops antibodies to part of itself. Gluten is found in wheat, barley and rye. The symptoms can be vague and coeliac disease is often missed as a diagnosis. In fact a colleague of mine who is an eminent surgeon missed the diagnosis in his own wife. In hindsight she had probably been suffering for a couple of years before the possibility of coeliac disease was discussed! It is relatively common, affecting one in a hundred people, but just like my colleague's wife, about three-quarters of those people don't yet know. That means there could be as many as half a million people in the UK today with coeliac disease who are yet to have a diagnosis!

Who gets coeliac disease?

Anyone can get coeliac disease but it is most common in people in their 40s and 50s. If you have a close relative with the diagnosis then you are more likely to suffer. You are also more likely to become coeliac if you have another autoimmune disease such as type 1 diabetes. We don't as yet know why some people develop this immune reaction.

How would I know if I had coeliac disease?

As I have already mentioned, the symptoms can be vague. They include fatigue, abdominal pain, bloating, flatulence and diarrhoea. Often these clues are missed until the disease has resulted in deficiencies of certain vitamins which may result in anaemia or mouth ulcers. In some patients, an intensely itchy rash develops called **dermatitis herpetiformis** and then the diagnosis is more obvious.

What should I do if I suspect I may have coeliac disease?

It will really help your doctor if you can keep a symptom and food diary, which should help to show whether your symptoms are related to gluten-containing foods such as bread, pasta and biscuits. Don't try to exclude these at this stage as if your doctor needs to arrange tests they will not show positive unless you are exposed to gluten at the time.

How is coeliac disease diagnosed?

In the past, the diagnosis was made by performing an endoscopy and taking a small biopsy of tissue from the lining of the small bowel. This was then examined under a microscope to look for the typical changes. The small bowel wall is lined with millions of tiny projections called **villi**. These massively increase the surface area of the gut and allow for improved absorption of nutrients. In gluten disease, these villi are flattened. Today we can do a blood test to look for antibodies called **endomysial antibodies** (EMA) and **transglutaminase antibodies**. If these are raised you will probably then be referred for the endoscopy and biopsy test, although not everyone will need this. In children with high levels of antibodies, for example, the doctors may make the diagnosis on blood tests alone. Not everyone with coeliac disease will test positive with blood tests so it is important that you go back to your doctor for further tests if your symptoms persist, even if your tests were normal. You will need to be exposed to gluten for at least one meal a day for six weeks prior to any tests for them to show positive. That's a tough one for some people as we are asking you to continue to have symptoms in order to make the diagnosis, but unfortunately that is the only way we can detect the antibodies.

How is coeliac disease treated?

Coeliac disease is managed by eliminating gluten from your diet for life. If you can do this, your symptoms should resolve in a small number of weeks, but most people find it difficult to know which foods contain gluten in the first instance. They are basically things like bread, pasta, cakes, pastries, biscuits and some cereals. Your GP will probably refer you to a dietician and in the early days you will find that you need to check food labels carefully. Unfortunately, if you eat gluten, your symptoms will recur. Some people with coeliac disease will develop symptoms on exposure to oats as well, but oats are fine for most sufferers. Your GP may also want you to take some supplements if other blood tests have shown you to be deficient in certain vitamins and minerals.

Are there any complications of coeliac disease?

As I have mentioned, untreated coeliac disease can lead to nutritional deficiencies so it is important that you stick to your diet. It can also be associated with an increased susceptibility to infection, so your doctor will offer you an annual flu jab and vaccination against other infections including haemophilus and pneumococcus. If you don't stick to your diet you could develop thin bones (**osteoporosis**) as a result of calcium deficiency. You may also develop other autoimmune conditions and there is a small increased risk that you may develop a type of lymphoma in the bowel wall later in life. If you stick to your diet these risks fall dramatically.

Small intestinal bacterial overgrowth (SIBO)

It is normal for the small intestine to contain bacteria. They are usually smaller in number and of a different type to the bacteria found in the large intestine. In SIBO, there are more bacteria than normal in the small intestine and there are more of the types generally seen in the large intestine.

Who gets SIBO?

Food is propelled through the gut with muscular contractions, and these contractions propel bacteria along with the food, thereby maintaining a smaller load of bacteria in the small gut. Conditions that affect the motility of the gut wall can result in SIBO. These include:

- diabetes mellitus
- scleroderma
- Crohn's disease (see Chapter 7)
- diverticular disease (see Chapter 7)
- previous bowel surgery.

What are the symptoms of SIBO?

The symptoms of SIBO can be very similar to coeliac disease and include abdominal pain, bloating, flatulence, and diarrhoea or constipation. If left undiagnosed the condition can mean that the bacteria compete for the nutrients in your food, meaning that fewer nutrients are absorbed into the system and patients may present with symptoms of deficiency.

How is SIBO diagnosed?

If your doctor suspects SIBO, he or she will arrange a hydrogen breath test. During this test you will be asked to fast for 12 hours. You will then be asked to inflate a balloon with a single long breath. After this, you will be given a known dose of a sugar, which is usually digested by bacteria found in the large colon. Repeat samples will be taken at regular intervals. We would normally expect to see a rise in hydrogen when the sugar reaches the large bowel but in SIBO there are two peaks as these bacteria are also present in the small bowel. The whole test takes around three hours. We can also culture bacteria from the small intestine using a tube passed through the nose and down the oesophagus, through the stomach and into the small intestine. Once in position a sample of intestinal fluid can be aspirated and analysed but this is a test that is more often used in research than in clinical practice.

How is SIBO treated?

Treatment usually involves a course of antibiotics but symptoms often recur after the antibiotics are stopped so this is combined with a long-term course of probiotics.

Protein-losing enteropathy

This is a condition where protein levels in the body are low because of a problem with the bowel. It can be caused by Crohn's disease (see Chapter 7), coeliac disease, some tumours and problems with the lymphatic system. If protein levels fall too low, then fluid leaks out of the blood vessels and may cause swollen ankles and fluid retention. The underlying cause should be treated.

Meckel's diverticulum

About two or three people in every hundred in the UK will have a Meckel's diverticulum and most will have no idea. It is a congenital abnormality (one that you are born with) and is a projection out of the wall of the ileum. About half contain some gastric tissue, which can produce stomach acid and may result in peptic ulceration. If symptoms develop the diverticulum can be surgically removed.

Carcinoid tumours

Carcinoid tumours are rare tumours that tend to occur in the over 60s. They are derived from what we call the neuroendocrine system and two-thirds of them occur in the digestive tract. The others start in the lung, kidney, ovary or testicle. We don't know why it happens but there does seem to be familial link, so if a close relative has had a carcinoid tumour, then you are slightly more at risk. It is more common in women and in people of African descent. Smoking and being very overweight can also increase your risk. There is also an association with diabetes and Zollinger-Ellison syndrome (see below) and other rare conditions including neurofibromatosis and tuberous sclerosis.

What are the symptoms of carcinoid?

In the early stages there may be no symptoms but as the tumour develops you may notice palpitations, flushing, wheezing, dizzy spells and diarrhoea.

How is carcinoid diagnosed?

If your GP suspects carcinoid, he or she will start by taking blood tests. Carcinoid tumours produce a chemical called **serotonin**, which is broken down to something called 5HIAA. If your blood level is raised, your doctor may then ask you to collect all your urine over a 24-hour period. 5HIAA is excreted in the urine, and high levels in a 24-hour collection suggest the presence of a carcinoid. While you are having the tests you will be asked to avoid foods rich in serotonin such as walnuts, bananas, avocados, pineapple and kiwi fruit. If these tests are positive you may then have other scans including barium studies, CT scans and MRI scans to locate the tumour. Your specialist may also look directly into the bowel with an endoscopy or colonoscopy.

How is carcinoid treated?

Once the carcinoid is located, you will then have other tests to check whether it has spread as this will influence what treatment you receive. If there is no spread and the tumour can be completely removed, you could be cured. Surgery is sometimes offered to relieve symptoms even if there is spread. Other treatments that you may be offered include radiotherapy and chemotherapy. Your specialist will discuss in detail with you which are likely to be appropriate for you and you should be involved in that decision-making. Don't be afraid to ask questions. It is important that you know what to expect from your treatment.

Zollinger-Ellison syndrome (ZES)

Zollinger-Ellison syndrome is a condition causing tumours and peptic ulcers in the gastrointestinal tract. The tumours are cancerous in about a quarter of patients.

What are the symptoms of ZES?

You may not have symptoms but if you do they can include fatigue, abdominal pain (often burning in nature), nausea, vomiting, diarrhoea and bleeding from the gastrointestinal tract.

How is ZES diagnosed?

If your doctor suspects ZES, he or she will arrange some blood tests looking for a substance called **gastrin**, which is produced by the tumours of ZES. If these levels are high, then you will probably be referred to a specialist for further tests including scans and endoscopies.

How is ZES treated?

The first thing your doctor will do is to switch off acid production by prescribing a course of a drug called a proton pump inhibitor. If you have developed an ulcer or the tumour is malignant, you will also need surgery.

Peutz-Jeghers syndrome

Peutz-Jeghers is an inherited condition. It is what we call autosomal dominant, which means that if your father or mother has the condition you have a 50 per cent chance of developing it too. It is rare but, unfortunately, it is associated with an increased risk of several cancers including cancer of the oesophagus, stomach, small and large bowel, thyroid, lung, womb and some types of breast cancer.

What are the symptoms of Peutz-Jeghers syndrome?

The classic giveaway sign is deep red- or purple-coloured spots around the lips. Occasionally these can also be found on the hands, feet and around the genitals. Other symptoms include recurrent abdominal pain and bleeding from the gut, usually due to the formation of polyps.

How is Peutz-Jeghers treated?

Unfortunately we can't cure the condition, but if you have Peutz-Jeghers syndrome you will be offered genetic counselling as any child of yours will have a 50 per cent chance of also having it. You will also be offered regular screening tests so that, should you develop cancer, it is detected early.

How to get an accurate diagnosis for small intestinal conditions

As you can see, so many of the small intestinal conditions I have discussed in this chapter produce very similar symptoms. In fact, gastrointestinal conditions can often be the most difficult to pin down in General Practice, particularly in the early stages, so before you go to see your doctor, take some time thinking about your symptoms. If you can tell your GP what flares your symptoms, when they seem to get better and what, if any, relationship there is between your diet and your symptoms, it will be clearer to your doctor and you will hopefully get a diagnosis sooner.

7

The large intestine

Constipation

Normal bowel movements are anything from twice a week to three times a day but the important thing is that you shouldn't need to strain to have your bowels open. If you are straining, you are becoming constipated and you should deal with things sooner rather than later.

Who gets constipated?

Anyone! It is particularly common in pregnancy and in older age but I have seen very young children really struggling with constipation too. It is more common if you are inactive and if you are becoming dehydrated. Diets that include a lot of processed foods will also predispose to constipation. Lots of medicines, especially painkillers, can cause constipation and some supplements such as iron or calcium supplements can also be to blame. Constipation can also be a symptom of other conditions including depression, an underactive thyroid, Parkinson's disease, irritable bowel syndrome, multiple sclerosis and diabetes. Rarely, it can also be due to a cancer in the bowel.

How do I know if I am constipated?

It's all about knowing what is normal for you. If you are someone who normally opens your bowels twice a day, then going twice a week could be constipated for you, whereas for someone else that may be their norm. If you are straining to open your bowels, passing very hard motions or feeling that you haven't completely emptied your rectum when you open your bowels then you are probably constipated. Sometimes, if you are very bunged up, you can get some leakage of watery faeces around the blockage, which is easy to mistake as diarrhoea.

How is constipation treated?

If you are prone to constipation, you should start by looking at your diet and lifestyle. Simply getting more active will encourage your bowels to be more active too. Increase your fluid intake and eat a well balanced diet rich in wholegrains, fruit and vegetables. If these measures don't help, you will need to consider a laxative. There are three main types.

- *Bulking agents*, such as ispaghula husk or methylcellulose. These are basically sources of extra fibre and work by bulking out the stool. They take a few days to work.
- *Osmotic laxatives*, such as lactulose and the macrogols. These work by increasing the amount of fluid in the motion so softening the stool. Again they can take several days to work.
- *Stimulant laxatives*, such as senna or bisacodyl. These work by stimulating the muscle in the bowel wall and should work overnight. They shouldn't be used long term as the bowel can start to rely on them.

What happens if constipation isn't treated?

If constipation is left untreated it can cause abdominal pain. There may be some leakage of liquid faeces around the blockage and as stools become harder and more difficult to pass, you could develop piles (see Chapter 8) or an anal fissure.

Diarrhoea

Diarrhoea is the passage of liquid or watery stools more frequently than usual. Common causes include:

- infection
- alcohol
- medicines
- irritable bowel syndrome
- inflammatory bowel disease
- neurological problems.

Most cases of diarrhoea will settle within a few days but it is important to drink plenty while you are suffering as it is easy to get dehydrated. People often ask me how much they should be drinking and it is impossible to be too prescriptive here as it depends on the severity of your diarrhoea. I advise people to keep an eye on the colour of their urine. Urine should be straw coloured, no darker. If your urine is darker than this then you are beginning to get dehydrated and you need to increase your fluid intake.

Do I need to see a doctor?

Most cases of diarrhoea will settle without the need to see your GP but you should seek medical advice if you:

- have travelled abroad recently;
- have been in hospital;
- suspect food poisoning;
- have blood in the diarrhoea;
- are becoming dehydrated;
- have symptoms that persist for more than four days.

What is the treatment for diarrhoea?

The mainstay of treatment is fluid. You can also buy rehy-dration sachets from the chemist to replace lost sugar and salt but don't be tempted to drink lots of high-sugar drinks as these can actually make things worse. Try to continue to eat little and often, sticking to bland foods until you are well. Don't take anti-diarrhoeal medicines in the early stages. Most cases of acute diarrhoea will be due to infection and your body needs to expel the bug from its system. However, diarrhoea means that you will be losing the good bacteria that help us digest our food too, so if your symptoms persist for more than a day or so, speak to your pharmacist about anti-diarrhoeal medication and you should consider a daily probiotic to top up your good bacteria. You should stay away from work until your symptoms have cleared for 48 hours to prevent spreading infection and take great care about hand washing after visiting the toilet and before handling food.

Clostridium difficile (C. diff)

Clostridium difficile is a bacteria that can live harmlessly in our gut as it is kept in check by the good bacteria that live in our bowels. We all have around 2 kilos of good bacteria, which help us digest our food. These are referred to as the gut flora. A course of antibiotics can alter the gut flora and allow *C. diff* to thrive, especially in the elderly and frail.

What are the symptoms of *C. diff*?

Watery diarrhoea following a course of antibiotics is the usual presentation. In some cases this can be very severe, leading to dehydration and inflammation of the gut lining called **pseudomembranous colitis**. This causes fever, bloody diarrhoea and abdominal pain.

How is *C. diff* diagnosed?

If you develop diarrhoea after a course of antibiotics or after a hospital stay, your GP may suspect *C. diff* and this can be confirmed by sending a stool sample to the laboratory to be analysed under a microscope. If you have had *C. diff* before you have an increased risk of a recurrence in the future.

How is C. diff treated?

Once the diagnosis is confirmed, your doctor will stop any antibiotics that you are currently taking and may start you on specific antibiotics aimed at killing the clostridium. Fluid replacement is vital. If you are very unwell you may be admitted to hospital and given fluids via a drip, but milder infections can be managed with fluids taken orally. It is important that you don't take anti-diarrhoeal medication as you need to allow the toxins produced by C. diff to clear from your body. Work is being done on faecal transplantation. Sounds gross, I know, but there are some really good results. The transplants are made from the faeces of household contacts because people who live in the same house and have roughly the same diet tend to have the same sort of gut flora. The faeces are mixed with saline solution and given to the patient via a nasogastric tube.

It is important to be fastidious about hygiene and hand washing to prevent spreading the disease to others.

Irritable bowel syndrome (IBS)

There has been much debate about whether sufferers of IBS have stronger than normal contractions of the muscular gut wall or a heightened awareness of normal contractions. To be honest, I suspect it is both. IBS is incredibly common, affecting about a third of us at some point in our lives.

How would I know if I had IBS?

IBS typically causes spasms of abdominal pain, which may be relieved by opening the bowels. It can cause diarrhoea or constipation and patients often describe a feeling of bloating and excess wind and a feeling that bowel movements are incomplete. This is called **tenesmus**. There may be mucus in the motions but IBS does not cause bleeding. IBS is a very individual disease. Some people get occasional

mild symptoms, while others find the condition truly debili-
tating. It is more common in women and there are a number
of triggers including:

- stress
- diet
- hormones.

How is IBS treated?

Your treatment will depend very much on how severe and
frequent your symptoms are. Start by keeping a symptom
diary for up to a month to see if you can identify a pattern to
your symptoms. It could be that they flare after eating certain
foods, around the time of your period, or when you are
under pressure and stressed. Identifying your triggers means
that you may be able to manage your symptoms simply by
avoiding certain foods or managing your diary so that you
don't put yourself under pressure around your period, for
example. If you are considering cutting out a whole food
group long term though, it is important that you speak to
a dietician to ensure that you replace the missing nutrients
with other foods. Common foods that seem to trigger a flare
include dairy products, wheat, rye, barley, onions, caffeine
and alcohol. IBS seems to be worse when we eat on the go, so
try to make time for proper meals and sit down to eat.

We always used to advise IBS sufferers to increase their
dietary fibre but research studies have shown mixed results.
Increasing fibre seems to help if symptoms are predominantly
that of constipation. But in IBS sufferers who experience diarrhoea, increasing fibre can actually make things worse. If you
are trying to increase your fibre intake, you should aim to
increase your soluble fibre; that is, oats, nuts, seeds and some
fruit and vegetables.

What is the low-FODMAP diet?

FODMAP stands for Fermentable Oligosaccharides, Disaccharides, Monosaccharides And Polyols. Cutting down on these foods helps some IBS sufferers but it's not an easy diet to stick to and you may need the help of a dietician to ensure that you are still getting a balanced diet. The sort of foods you will need to cut back on include dairy products; green vegetables, such as peas, sprouts, broccoli and cabbage; artificial sweeteners; and fruits such as peaches, nectarines, apples and cherries.

Are probiotics useful for IBS?

The idea behind taking probiotics is that they boost levels of good bacteria and aid digestion. Some of my patients have found taking a daily probiotic very helpful in managing their IBS, but they don't seem to work for everyone. My line is that they are well worth a try and you need to do it for at least a month. Keep a symptom diary during that time so that you can see if there has been a difference and if you're not convinced, it might be worth trying a different one for another month.

Are there any medications for treating IBS?

Yes, lots! I use antispasmodics to relieve spasm in the muscular gut wall. There are several different types so don't despair if you don't get a result straight away – go back to your GP and he or she will try an alternative. Peppermint capsules are good for bloating and an old fashioned antidepressant called **amitriptyline** can also improve symptoms.

Are there alternative treatments for IBS?

Stress plays a big role in flare ups of IBS symptoms, so anything that helps you relax and manage stress is worth a try. I know that many of my patients have found great relief from hypnotherapy and cognitive behavioural therapy. Some studies have also shown a benefit of using Chinese herbal remedies too.

Is there any link between IBS and bowel cancer?

No. Patients are often worried about long-term implications of having IBS but there is no link with cancer at all.

Inflammatory bowel disease (IBD)

Inflammatory bowel disease is the term used for a group of conditions causing inflammation along the digestive tract. The two most common forms and the ones I will discuss here are Crohn's disease and ulcerative colitis (UC).

Crohn's disease

Crohn's disease can affect any part of the gut from the mouth to the anus. There are about 115,000 people in the UK currently living with Crohn's. It usually presents in your late teens or twenties and affects more women than men. We don't know exactly what causes Crohn's but there does appear to be a genetic component. One theory is that an infection may trigger an immune response in the genetically predisposed. The combined contraceptive pill and non-steroidal anti-inflammatory drugs may also trigger it. It is also more common in smokers.

How would I know if I had Crohn's?

Symptoms vary from person to person depending on which part of the gastrointestinal tract is involved and how extensive the disease is. Most patients will experience a combination of these symptoms:

- diarrhoea (there may be mucus or blood in the diarrhoea)
- abdominal pain
- weight loss
- fatigue
- mouth ulcers.

If large areas of the small intestine are involved, then patients may also show signs of nutritional deficiency because nutrients are not being properly absorbed. The typical pattern is that patients experience flare ups and then times of remission.

Crohn's disease can lead to narrowing of the lumen (the inside) of the gut called strictures. The inflammation can also break through the bowel wall causing a perforation and sometimes the inflammation can cause a channel between two parts of the body. This is called a **fistula** and sometimes they can form between the bowel and the skin around the anus or vagina, meaning faeces leak uncontrollably. There is also a small increased risk of bowel cancer in Crohn's sufferers.

How is Crohn's diagnosed?

Crohn's disease is usually diagnosed following a colonoscopy, where biopsies can be taken. The lining of the intestine looks pink and smooth to the naked eye but in Crohn's disease there are patches of the gut lining that look like cobblestones and the appearance under the microscope will confirm the diagnosis. You may also have blood tests looking for particular proteins that are raised in inflammatory diseases.

How is Crohn's treated?

Mild flare ups may require no treatment, but more significant symptoms will usually be treated with steroids in the first instance. These can be given by mouth, by enema or by injection depending on which part of the intestine is involved and the severity of the flare.

More severe disease may require medicines to suppress the immune system such as azathioprine, methotrexate and mercaptopurine or genetically engineered antibodies called monoclonal antibodies. These stronger drugs are usually started by a specialist and need regular monitoring. Your doctor will check with blood tests to see if you are becoming deficient in certain nutrients and will advise on supplements if any of these tests show a deficiency. Surgery is sometimes needed to treat complications such as fistulas and strictures or to remove whole areas of severely affected gut.

Ulcerative colitis

Ulcerative colitis (UC) is very similar to Crohn's disease and symptoms may present in a similar way. It affects about two in every thousand people in the UK and usually presents between puberty and middle age. It differs from Crohn's in that only the large bowel is affected and, as its name implies, it causes ulceration rather than the cobblestone appearance of Crohn's; the inflammation is confined to the superficial layer of the gut lining so there is not the same risk of perforation and fistula formation. UC is one of the few conditions that is more common in non-smokers than smokers. Just like Crohn's we don't really know what causes UC, but we do know that about 20 per cent of UC sufferers have a close relative with the condition so there does seem to be a genetic link and again there is a theory that UC could be triggered by an infection in the genetically susceptible. And, as with Crohn's, UC sufferers have a slight increase risk of developing bowel cancer.

How can I tell the difference between UC and Crohn's?

You probably couldn't. Flare ups of both conditions are very similar and generally present with abdominal pain, bloody diarrhoea and fatigue. The diagnosis is made on colonoscopy and biopsy.

How is UC treated?

Treatment of UC is very similar to that of Crohn's with one notable exception. In UC we are more likely to use a group of drugs called the aminosalicylates, which can be taken by mouth or by enema to counter the way inflammation develops in UC.

Are there other complications of inflammatory bowel disease?

Patients with inflammatory bowel disease may experience symptoms outside of the gastrointestinal tract and these include:

- inflammation in the eyes
- arthritis
- ankylosing spondylitis (an inflammatory arthritis of the spine)
- skin rashes
- liver problems
- gallstones
- kidney stones
- blood clots.

Diverticular disease

In diverticular disease, there are small bulges in the gut wall. These are common and may be associated with mild abdominal pain, bloating and rectal bleeding, but in most cases they cause no problem at all until they become infected, which is referred to as **diverticulitis**. Diverticulitis develops in about a quarter of people with diverticular disease (also sometimes referred to as **diverticulosis**). Diverticulitis may be associated with more severe abdominal pain, diarrhoea and a fever.

Who gets diverticulitis?

Diverticular disease is more common in the elderly. It is also more common in the Western world and it is thought this may be related to our diet. In some cases there is a family history of the condition; whether this is linked to common diets or genetics is not yet clear. Other risk factors include:

- obesity
- constipation
- smoking
- taking non-steroidal anti-inflammatory drugs, such as ibu-profen or aspirin.

How is diverticular disease diagnosed?

If your doctor suspects diverticular disease, he or she will probably arrange for you to have a colonoscopy and or a CT scan. For either of these you will need to take a strong laxative the night before, so make sure you are close to a toilet. If you need a CT scan for suspected diverticulosis, you will have a tube inserted into the rectum so that air can be pumped in.

How is diverticular disease treated?

Over the counter painkillers are usually sufficient to control the pain of diverticular disease and you may need a regular laxative to prevent constipation. Stool softeners and bulk-forming agents are better than stimulant laxatives in this instance. Diverticulitis will need a course of antibiotics and your GP may recommend you stick to a fluid diet for a couple of days. You will then be advised to stick to a low fibre diet (rather than the usual high fibre diet) to reduce the amount of faeces you produce while the inflammation settles. In severe cases of diverticulitis, you may need hospital admission for intravenous antibiotics and feeding while the bowel recovers.

Can diverticular disease cause other problems?

Most people with diverticular disease don't develop other problems. I am often asked if there is an associated risk of bowel cancer and the answer is no. Occasionally patients with severe disease may develop an abscess or fistula, which can lead to peritonitis. Recurrent infection can also lead to scarring which may cause intestinal obstruction. These sort of complications are not common but if they occur, they often require surgery and some patients with severe disease may end up needing a colostomy bag.

What can I do to help myself?

It is important that you drink plenty of fluid and stick to a high fibre diet rich in fruit and vegetables. Some people find that nuts and seeds cause flare up, the theory being that they get stuck in the diverticula and act as a focus for infection. If this is you, then try to avoid them in your diet. Some of my patients find taking a daily probiotic to aid digestion has helped. If despite these measures you are still prone to constipation, speak to your pharmacist about the best type of laxative for you.

Colonic polyps

Colonic polyps are small cells that form on the lining of the colon. They are benign, but a small percentage of them can become cancerous, so if they are found, they are usually removed.

Who gets colonic polyps?

Anyone can develop polyps but they are more common in the over 50s, the obese and in smokers. There are also two inherited conditions, familial adenomatous polyposis (FAP) and Lynch syndrome. If you have either of these conditions, your children will have a 50 per cent chance of inheriting the same condition. Both these conditions cause multiple polyps that can first develop in the teens, so require regular colonoscopies to check for new polyps, which can then be removed. They are also more common in patients with inflammatory bowel disease and patients with poorly controlled type 2 diabetes.

How would I know if I had polyps?

Often colonic polyps cause no symptoms at all but if they do, most commonly it is rectal bleeding. This can be in the form of fresh blood in the stool or a black tarry consistency to the stool if the bleeding is from higher up in the bowel. Sometimes they can cause abdominal pain or a change in your bowel habit, which could be towards constipation or diarrhoea.

How are polyps diagnosed?

Polyps are usually diagnosed with a colonoscopy. Occasionally they are diagnosed using a CT scan.

How are polyps treated?

Polyps can only be treated by physically removing them. This can usually be done at the time of colonoscopy by using forceps or a wire loop to snare the polyp. If you have one of the rare inherited conditions associated with polyps and have multiple polyps, your specialist may suggest you have part of your bowel removed.

Colorectal cancer

Colon cancer is the fourth most common cancer in the UK

Who gets colon cancer?

Eighty per cent of bowel cancers occur in the over 60s. About 5 per cent are due to inherited conditions such as FAP or Lynch syndrome. Other risk factors include:

- polyps
- Crohn's disease and ulcerative colitis
- diabetes
- testicular cancer
- womb cancer
- lymphoma

- dietary factors (see below)
- excess alcohol.

How would I know if I had colon cancer?

In the early stages you may have no symptoms at all, which is why we offer screening to those at risk, because like all cancers, the earlier colon cancer is diagnosed, the better the outlook. When symptoms develop they can include:

- bleeding from the rectum or in the stool
- abdominal pain
- change in bowel habit, which can be towards constipation or diarrhoea
- unexplained weight loss
- a lump in the abdomen
- symptoms of anaemia as a result of blood loss.

If you develop these symptoms it is important that you see your GP straight away.

How is colon cancer diagnosed?

If your GP suspects colon cancer he or she will refer you to have a colonoscopy urgently, and you should receive that appointment within two weeks. If there is anything suspicious to be seen on colonoscopy, the specialist will take biopsies to be analysed under a microscope and if cancer is confirmed, then you will have further tests to see if the cancer has spread.

How is colon cancer treated?

If colon cancer is found early it can be cured by surgery. If it has spread you may also need a combination of radiotherapy and chemotherapy.

What can I do to reduce my risk of developing colon cancer?

We know that a high fibre diet protects from colon cancer so try to incorporate plenty of fruit and vegetables into your diet – at least five portions a day (see below). Eating a lot of red meat, especially processed meat, increases your risk so keep this to a minimum, but eating fish probably reduces your risk. Diets high in calcium probably also lower the risk of developing bowel cancer. Obesity increases your risk so try to maintain a health BMI between 18.5 and 25. You can calculate your BMI by dividing your weight in kilos by the square of your height in metres:

BMI = weight in kilos divided by
(height in metres × height in metres)

Excess alcohol also increases your risk so keep to recommended limits (see Chapter 10). Take regular exercise and don't smoke as this will reduce your risk. Studies have also shown that taking a daily low dose aspirin protects against colon cancer but discuss this with your doctor first as aspirin can cause side effects which may mean it is not appropriate for you. Hormone replacement therapy and the combined contraceptive pill may also be protective.

What is a portion of fruit or vegetables?

A portion of fruit or vegetables is about 80 grams of fresh produce or 30 grams of dried. As a guideline this is:

- 1 apple, orange, banana or medium-sized tomato;
- 2 plums, kiwi fruit, satsumas or broccoli spears;
- ½ a grapefruit;
- a slice of pineapple or melon;
- 3 heaped tablespoons of peas, sweetcorn or beans;
- 7 cherry tomatoes.

Tinned or frozen fruit and vegetables count and fruit juice

counts, but only as one portion. If you drank more than one glass of orange juice for example, it would still only count as one portion because there is less fibre in juice. Potatoes don't count as a vegetable in this instance.

Can I be screened for colon cancer?

If you are registered with an NHS GP in England and are between 60 and 69, you will be offered bowel screening in the form of a testing kit that you will be sent in the post. The screening programme includes people up to 74 in Scotland and Wales and starts at 50 in Wales. There are plans to extend the screening programme so that everyone in the UK will be offered the test between the ages of 50 and 74. The test involves smearing a small sample of your poo onto a test card, which is then sent back to be analysed in the laboratory for microscopic traces of blood. It may not sound much like fun, but it is a simple test that literally could save your life. If the samples test positive for blood, you will then be offered a colonoscopy. There are plans to include a one-off sigmoid-oscopy for everyone over 55. You may also be screened if you:

- have had bowel cancer before;
- have had polyps;
- have FAP or Lynch syndrome;
- have several relatives with bowel cancer;
- have Crohn's disease or ulcerative colitis.

Appendicitis

The appendix is a finger-like projection at the junction of the small and large intestine. When it gets inflamed it is called appendicitis.

Who gets appendicitis?

Appendicitis is common – one in 13 of us will have it and I'm one of them! In fact if I hadn't had appendicitis I might never have become a doctor. It was while recuperating from my surgery that I first became fascinated by medicine. Around 40,000 people will be admitted to hospital with appendicitis this year. It is most common in 10 to 20 year olds but can occur later in life.

What are the symptoms of appendicitis?

Appendicitis starts as a pain in the middle of your abdomen, which moves to the lower right hand side over a period of hours. The area becomes very tender to touch. It is usually associated with a fever, loss of appetite and nausea. You may also develop diarrhoea and moving about becomes very painful so patients want to lie still.

How is appendicitis treated?

In most cases the appendix will need to be surgically removed and this is usually done by keyhole surgery (laparoscopy) today, which means that you will be back to normal within a couple of weeks. Occasionally surgeons can't remove the appendix laparoscopically, in which case open surgery is needed and recovery is likely to be nearer six weeks. If surgery is delayed there is a risk of the appendix bursting and causing peritonitis (infection in the abdominal cavity), which can be life threatening.

Hernias

Hernias occur when there is a weakness in the abdominal wall and part of the bowel pushes through. There are several different types.

- *Inguinal hernias* These are found in the groin. They are more common in men because there is a natural weakness where the testicles descend from inside the abdomen into the scrotum.

- *Femoral hernias* These are also found in the groin but are much less common and are more frequently seen in women.
- *Umbilical hernias* These are usually seen in babies when the opening for the umbilical cord hasn't healed completely.
- *Hiatus hernias* See Chapter 5.
- *Incisional hernias* These occur as a result of weakness created by surgery.

Once a hernia has formed it won't repair itself without surgery but not all hernias require an operation. The decision on whether or not to operate will depend on the size of the hernia, the impact that it has on your quality of life and your general health. Interestingly, large hernias are usually less of a worry as they can easily be 'reduced', which means pushed back inside. Smaller hernias can sometimes get stuck out. This is called strangulated and can lead to **necrosis** (death) of the tissue, so needs urgent surgery.

How would I know if a hernia was strangulating?

If you develop sudden severe pain and the hernia is tender to touch and you are vomiting or unable to pass stools, this may mean your hernia is strangulating and you should seek urgent medical advice.

Faecal incontinence

It is estimated that at some point in their lives one in ten people will experience faecal incontinence, where there is an involuntary leakage of stool. For most people it may be a very occasional leak, for example, during a bout of infective diarrhoea, but for others it is a persistent and very distressing problem.

What causes faecal incontinence?

Most cases will be as a result of diarrhoea or, the opposite, when there is leakage of liquid faeces around a blockage caused by constipation. It can also occur because of damage to the nerves after surgery or due to neurological diseases such as spinal injury or multiple sclerosis. It is also seen in dementia. The treatment will depend on the cause.

8
The anus

Haemorrhoids

Haemorrhoids are swollen blood vessels, like varicose veins, around the rectum. They can be visible outside the anus (external) or inside where they can't be seen (internal).

Who gets haemorrhoids?

Anyone can get haemorrhoids. In fact about half of us will at some point in our lives. They are more common as we get older and are particularly a problem for overweight people and pregnant women. Anything that causes increased abdominal pressure will increase the risk of developing them, so people who strain to open their bowels, those with a chronic cough, persistent vomiting or who sit for long periods of time. Like most old wives' tales, there is some truth in the belief that sitting on cold seats will give you piles. In fact it has nothing to do with the temperature of the seat but simply sitting for long periods is the risk. Diet undoubtedly plays a role as well. A diet high in processed food with little fibre will make you prone to constipation and may lead to haemorrhoids.

What are the symptoms of haemorrhoids?

There may be no symptoms at all. Internal piles that are higher up in the rectum, for example, cause no pain and cannot be seen without a proctoscope. The most common symptom is fresh red blood when opening your bowels, either seen on the toilet paper after wiping yourself or in the pan. It is separate from the stool. You might be aware of a lump hanging down outside your anus with external piles and the skin around the anus may feel itchy and irritated. They are not usually painful unless they become strangulated. This happens when the blood supply is cut off to piles that protrude outside the body and can be intensely painful. Occasionally a clot may form in the pile, which again is extremely painful and takes a few days to resolve.

How are haemorrhoids diagnosed?

External piles can be easily seen with the naked eye and your doctor will make the diagnosis after looking at your anus. He will ask you to lie on your left side with your knees curled up like a baby so that he or she can easily see your rectum and he or she may need to insert a finger into your rectum to feel for any other piles or abnormalities. He will need to use a small instrument called a proctoscope to look higher up into the rectum to check for internal piles.

What is the treatment for haemorrhoids?

First-line treatment is to use creams and/or pessaries to shrink the piles. If this is not helping or the piles are very prominent, your doctor may suggest a number of options including:

- Banding – small elastic bands are placed around the base of the piles to cut off the blood supply and a few days later the haemorrhoid drops off. It's exactly the same as the procedure farmers use to castrate lambs and remove their long tails!
- Injection – phenol can be injected into haemorrhoids, which then shrivel up.
- Haemorrhoidectomy – a surgeon can physically cut out the piles.

Some doctors also use electric current, heat or infrared energy to remove haemorrhoids.

What can I do to prevent them recurring?

The most important thing you can do is to keep your stools soft so that you don't strain to have your bowels open, so make sure you drink plenty of fluid and eat a high fibre diet including lots of fruit and vegetables. Few people realize that our bowels often reflect our activity so the more sedentary you are, the more sluggish your bowels are likely to be. Avoid sitting for long periods and try to be as active as you can to keep your bowels moving.

Anal fissure

An anal fissure is a tear in the delicate skin around the anus. They are relatively common and cause a sharp pain when trying to open your bowels or fresh bleeding from the back passage. They often occur as a result of constipation and because bowel movements are painful, some people try to avoid opening their bowels, which only makes things worse.

How are anal fissures treated?

Most anal fissures will heal on their own and really it's a case of making sure that you avoid constipation and keep your stool soft with changes to your diet and lifestyle (see Chapter 7). If they are very sore, your GP may prescribe some local anaesthetic cream. An ointment of glyceryl trinitrate improves blood supply to the area and therefore promotes healing. Rarely, surgery is needed.

Pruritus ani

Pruritus ani simply means an itchy bottom. It is more common in men than women and tends to occur in middle age. It is also more common in people with a lot of hair around the bottom and in those who sweat more.

What causes pruritus ani?

In about half of all cases, pruritus ani is due to skin conditions such as psoriasis, eczema or lichen sclerosis. In the other half, the cause may not be immediately obvious but common triggers include:

- diarrhoea
- irritation from soaps, perfumed products or the dye in coloured toilet paper
- thrush
- worms
- scabies
- haemorrhoids
- citrus fruits, tomatoes and spicy foods
- tea, coffee, milk and beer.

How is pruritus ani treated?

The treatment will depend on the cause. If there is an underlying skin problem then your doctor will treat that and your symptoms should resolve. The problem is that it is easy to get into a vicious itch–scratch cycle. When you feel the itch, you have the urge to scratch, which temporarily relieves the symptoms but scratching traumatizes the skin, which in turn exacerbates the itch.

If you are struggling with pruritus ani, make sure you keep your fingernails short so that you don't damage the skin when you are half asleep. You can also buy cotton mittens from the chemist to wear at night. Avoid all perfumed products and only use soft white tissue paper. Wash around your anus with water only and pat the skin dry. Change your underwear daily and avoid synthetic fabrics as these are likely to make you sweat more, which can irritate the skin. Keep a food diary and if you think a particular food is making the problem worse, then try cutting it out for a while to see if this helps. You could also try taking an antihistamine at night to relieve the itch.

In some cases I have used a low dose of an antidepressant called amitriptyline with good effect.

Pilonidal sinus

A pilonidal sinus is a small tract that forms between the deep tissues around the anus and the skin. The word pilonidal actually means 'nest of hairs' and usually the sinus starts with hair getting stuck under the skin causing inflammation and ultimately infection.

Who gets pilonidal sinuses?

Pilonidal sinuses are more common in men and in those with a lot of dark body hair. (Dark hair tends to be tougher and more able to bury into the skin). Obesity and a sedentary lifestyle also increase the risk. The condition sometimes runs in families, which may be due to an inherited abnormality in the skin around the buttocks.

How would I know if I had a pilonidal sinus?

There may not be much to see but you will notice increasing pain, particularly when sitting down, and then there may be some swelling. Ultimately the infection may burst through the skin and you will notice pus around the area. When this happens there is less pressure and so it will feel less painful but it is important that you seek medical help as it is unlikely the infection will heal properly without surgery.

What does the surgery involve?

There are various operations available but the idea is to excise all the infected tissue and the sinus. Often the wound is not stitched up as in most operations but is left open and dressed daily to allow the wound to heal from the bottom up and hopefully prevent the problem recurring. It takes several weeks to heal. If the sinus is very extensive or if there are problems with recurrence you may need plastic surgery to the area.

What can I do to prevent a sinus recurring?

If you have had a pilonidal sinus there is always the risk of recurrence so try to maintain a healthy body weight and avoid sitting for long periods of time if you can. You may also be advised to remove excess body hair from the area.

9

The pancreas

Diabetes

In this chapter when I talk about diabetes I will refer to diabetes mellitus. Diabetes insipidus is a different condition where you have problems controlling the balance of water in your body. Like diabetes mellitus it can make you excessively thirsty but it is not linked to being overweight or obese. It is due to a problem either in the brain or in the kidneys.

There are two types of diabetes mellitus. Type 2 is by far the more common type, accounting for 90 to 95 per cent of all adult diabetics and is usually related to excess weight. Type 1 diabetes is not linked to weight. It is a condition where your body develops antibodies to the beta cells in your pancreas. These are the cells that produce insulin and very quickly your insulin levels drop.

Type 1 diabetes

Type 1 diabetes usually appears in younger people and often in children.

What causes type 1 diabetes?

Type 1 diabetes is a disorder of the immune system, where the body produces antibodies to its own pancreas and stops the production of insulin. We are not sure why this happens but researchers are looking into the possibility that is triggered by a virus in those that are susceptible. There is also a genetic component in that it does seem to run in families.

What are the symptoms of type 1 diabetes?

The most common symptoms are of feeling excessively thirsty and passing more urine. You may also feel very tired and lethargic and tend to lose weight unexpectedly. You may notice that you get recurrent infections, particularly recurrent thrush, and that any wounds are slower to heal. There can also be blurred vision as the lens of the eye changes shape. If left undiagnosed and blood sugar levels are allowed to run very high, you may vomit and develop fruity-smelling breath. This may be associated with abdominal pain and is a medical emergency. If sugar levels are allowed to continue to rise unchecked it can ultimately cause a fit or coma so get medical help without delay!

How is type 1 diabetes diagnosed?

A simple blood test will show if your sugar levels are high; if your blood sugar is greater than 11.1 mmol/litre then a diagnosis is made straight away. It is the same if a fasting sample is greater than 7 mmol/litre. If your sugar level is high but not this high, you will be asked to do something called a **glucose tolerance test** (GTT – see below). Another blood test called the **glycated haemoglobin** (HbA1c) gives us an idea of how well blood sugar levels have been controlled in recent weeks. If it is greater than 6.5 per cent this is also diagnostic of diabetes and the HbA1c test is also used to monitor diabetes after diagnosis.

How is type 1 diabetes treated?

Insulin can be given as individual injections and there are many different types. Some are short-acting, meaning their effect doesn't last long, some have intermediate action and some are long-acting. You may well need a combination of different types. Insulin can also be given via a pump, which means fewer injections. If you are injecting regularly you will be advised to rotate your injection sites as repeated injections at the same site will be uncomfortable and can cause changes in the underlying fatty tissue. This is called **lipodystrophy** and looks like dimples and lumps under the skin. You will also need to follow a diet and lifestyle like that described below for type 2 diabetics.

Type 2 diabetes

Type 2 diabetes used to also be called adult onset or maturity onset diabetes because it was seen in older people generally over 40. These alternative names have now been dropped because that is not the case. Type 2 diabetes is usually linked to being overweight and, sadly, because we are becoming bigger as a nation and lots of young people are now clinically obese we are seeing type 2 diabetes in young adults and even in children. Unlike type 1 diabetes, type 2 diabetes develops slowly. If it is picked up early then often it can be managed with diet and lifestyle changes alone but if left untreated will need prescription medication and ultimately some type 2 diabetics will need insulin by injection. Type 2 diabetes develops either because you have become resistant to the effect of insulin, so normal insulin levels just aren't enough to keep your blood sugar under control, or your body doesn't make enough insulin. In some cases it can be a mixture of both.

Who gets type 2 diabetes?

More people than you think! It is estimated that in the UK alone while you are reading this, there are 750,000 people walking around getting on with their day to day life who have diabetes and have no idea. Because the symptoms can be vague (see below) and come on so insidiously, it is perfectly possible to have the condition and not be aware that you are unwell. There are several risk factors for type 2 diabetes:

- *Weight* Being clinically overweight (BMI 25–30) or clinically obese (BMI over 30) significantly increases your risk and most type 2 diabetics are overweight.
- *Waist circumference* Women with waist circumferences of greater than 80 cm (31.5 inches) and men with waist circumferences greater than 94 cm (37 inches), or 90 cm (35.5 inches) if you are of Asian or Afro Caribbean descent, are at increased risk.
- *Ethnicity* The different risk for waist circumference above is because type 2 diabetes is about five times more common in people of Asian and Afro Caribbean descent.
- *Family history* If your mother, father, brother, sister or child has diabetes you are more likely to develop the condition.
- *Impaired glucose tolerance* If it is found on routine testing that you have a slightly raised glucose level which is not high enough to make a diagnosis of diabetes but is higher than normal, you will be asked to have what is called a glucose tolerance test. This involves having nothing to eat or drink for 8 or 12 hours. You will then have a blood test which is referred to as the 'fasting sample'. Then, you will be given a sugary drink containing a known amount of glucose and blood samples are taken again at given intervals to see how your body manages that known amount of sugar. If your body struggles to get your blood sugar level back to the normal range then this is called impaired glucose tolerance and puts you at increased risk of developing type 2 diabetes.
- *Pregnancy* If you have impaired glucose tolerance or became diabetic during pregnancy this usually resolves after the baby is born, but it does increase your risk of developing type 2 diabetes later in life.

How is type 2 diabetes diagnosed?

The symptoms of type 2 diabetes are vague and come on slowly. You may experience lethargy and increased thirst. You may find that you are passing urine more frequently and you may have recurrent infections such as thrush but because they develop slowly over many, many months a lot of people don't really notice, so most cases of type 2 diabetes are picked up after routine health checks.

In the first instance your doctor may notice there is sugar in your urine, which is picked up on urine dipstick testing. If this is found you will be asked to have a blood test, usually on a fasting sample. That means having nothing to eat or drink for several hours (usually about eight hours, so in most instances this would mean overnight) before your blood test. Fasting blood sugar levels should be between 3.6 mmol/litre and 6.1 mmol/litre. If fasting sugar levels are higher than 7 mmol/litre or if what we call a 'random glucose level', i.e. one taken at any time of the day, is greater than 11.1 mmol/litre, this is diagnostic of diabetes. If an individual has no symptoms but the abnormality is picked up on routine testing, then we repeat the tests to confirm the diagnosis but one test is enough for diagnosis if a person has symptoms of type 2 diabetes.

How is type 2 diabetes managed?

In the first instance you will probably be asked to have an appointment with the practice nurse to talk through what you can do to change your diet and lifestyle. For some, lifestyle changes alone may be all that is needed but it is important that you know exactly what you can and can't eat. It may feel daunting at first but to be honest much of what I have already said in this book will be relevant to you. While you are waiting for that appointment, try to keep a food diary so that the nurse (and you!) can see where you are going wrong and give you some tips on how you manage this going forward. You will need to adopt a low fat, salt and sugar diet. Low fat because managing your weight is crucial, low salt because having diabetes means you are prone to high blood pressure and kidney problems and low sugar because by definition, having diabetes means difficulty handling and processing sugar and, of course, low sugar will help keep your weight under control too.

This is a rough guide to the diet you should aim for:

- *Total fat less than 35 per cent of total calorie intake.* This can be achieved by limiting fried or processed foods and high fat snacks such as crisps, cake and biscuits.
- *Trans fats and saturated fats should constitute only a third of your total fat intake.*
- *Total carbohydrates 40–60 per cent of total calorie intake.* It's tough but this means being careful with fizzy drinks, squashes and cordials, limiting cakes and biscuits, and opting for foods with a low glycaemic index. This simply means those that produce less of a peak in blood sugar levels. So, for example, the blood sugar peak seen after eating pasta is much lower than that after eating chips. Pasta has a lower glycaemic index than potato.

Not everyone with type 2 diabetes is overweight but the majority are, and tackling this will be a priority for you. It is likely to be a long haul but even modest weight loss can make a real difference. Depending on the blood results, your GP and nurse may suggest that you look at lifestyle changes alone for a few months. If they can see your HbA1c returning to normal as a result of these changes then you may not need to do anything further.

What if my blood tests remain abnormal?

If your blood tests remain abnormal despite making changes to your lifestyle, your doctor will prescribe medication to help bring your blood sugar levels under control. It is important that you persevere with lifestyle changes, as even if you need medication now, as you continue to bring your weight down and improve your fitness you may find that you will be able to come off your medication. Although, as I have said

before, don't ever be tempted to try this without the help of
your doctor. There are several types of tablets used to keep
blood sugar levels under control:

- *Metformin* The drug metformin is a biguanide. It improves
  sensitivity to insulin and may help with weight loss. It
  is the first drug we use in type 2 diabetes associated with
  weight issues since most, although not all, type 2 diabetics
  are overweight.
- *Nateglinide and repaglinide* These drugs stimulate the release
  of insulin. They work very quickly after being taken but
  they don't last for long so they are taken immediately
  before eating. Nateglinide is only licensed to be used in
  conjunction with metformin but repaglinide can be used
  on its own in type 2 diabetics who are not overweight or
  who cannot tolerate metformin.
- *Sulfonylureas* These drugs work by enhancing insulin secretion so by definition they are only useful if the pancreas is
  capable of producing some insulin. There are different sulfonylureas and which one you are described will depend
  on your individual circumstances. They have different
  lengths of action – some of the more long acting types
  may mean that you are at risk of becoming hypogly-
  caemic. That means your blood sugar falls too low. This
  can be a medical emergency so your doctor will fine-tune
  which particular sulfonylurea is best for you. The sulfonylureas include glibenclamide, gliclazide, glimepiride,
  glipizide and tolbutamide.
- *Pioglitazone* This drug works by reducing insulin resist-
  ance. It can be used on its own or alongside metformin or
  a sulfonylurea but it must be used with care. It has been
  shown to increase the risk of heart failure when combined
  with insulin so shouldn't be used in anyone with known
  heart failure and all patients who take this drug need to be
  closely monitored.
- *Gliptins* These drugs increase insulin secretion and reduce

glucagon secretion. Glucagon is another pancreatic hormone which works to raise blood sugar levels when they start to fall. They can be used on their own or in conjunction with metformin or a sulfonylurea, or with pioglitazone. They include saxagliptin, sitagliptin and vildagliptin.

- *Acarbose* This drug delays the digestion and absorption of carbohydrate and sugar from the gut. It is generally reserved for those patients who cannot tolerate other anti-diabetic medication.

What if tablets can't control my type 2 diabetes?

If you have tried lifestyle changes and despite adding in tablets, your sugar levels and HbA1c levels remain abnormal your doctor will suggest you try injections. There are two main types of injection therapy:

- *Insulin* See type 1 diabetes.
- *Exenatide and liraglutide* These drugs increase insulin secretion, reduce glucagon secretion and delay gastric emptying so that there is a slower delivery of food to the small intestine where the sugar is absorbed.

Will I need other medication?

If you have diabetes, whether it is type 1 or type 2, your risks of developing high blood pressure, high cholesterol and heart disease amongst other things, increases. Your doctor will want to monitor you for these problems and will advise on whether you need medication. The good news through all of this, though, is that if you persevere with your lifestyle changes you could potentially, under the supervision of your medical team, come off all the medicines. That is quite some incentive!

How will my diabetes be monitored?

Having diabetes means that you will need regular review at their GP surgeries and, maybe, also at the hospital. You will need blood tests to check your glucose levels and your HbA1c and you will also need cholesterol blood tests and tests to check your kidney function. You will have your eyes checked every year as diabetes can affect your vision and you will have regular blood pressure checks and checks on your sensation and your feet. It is important that whenever you have an appointment that you leave knowing when the next one will be and whether it is down to you to make a note of when to go back or whether you will be called.

Why is it so important to control my sugar level when I don't feel unwell with it?

You may feel totally well with higher than normal blood sugar levels but persistently high glucose levels in the blood damages the blood vessels, the body's organs and the nerves. In real terms this means that if you ignore your condition you are at significant risk of some serious health issues in the future. These include the problems outlined below.

Heart disease and stroke

If you have diabetes, you are up to five times more likely to have a heart attack or stroke because they are more likely to develop furring of the arteries. This could present as angina where classically you experience a crushing central chest pain on exertion or after eating a meal. The pain sometimes radiates to the jaw or the left arm and may be associated with shortness of breath and nausea. Pain like this should never be ignored and needs urgent medical attention. If the pain persists it could indicate that you are having a heart attack and need to call an ambulance immediately. A stroke may present as slurring of your speech, droop on one side of your face or weakness in your arms and or legs.

High blood pressure

People with diabetes are more prone to high blood pressure as the arteries become narrower. It is completely normal for anyone's blood pressure to go up when they are anxious, in pain or exercising but if blood pressure is consistently raised this puts a strain on your heart. I liken it to driving a car. If you put your foot on the throttle occasionally to accelerate past an obstacle, your car will cope perfectly well, but if you drive around constantly with your foot on the floor, it won't be long before the engine starts to struggle. If your arteries are narrowed and the same volume of blood needs to be pumped around by your heart then it stands to reason that your heart is having to work harder to force the blood around your body.

High cholesterol

Having diabetes increases the risk of high cholesterol and your doctor will be keen to keep your cholesterol levels lower than if you did not have diabetes.

Visual problems

Poor diabetic control can make the small blood vessels that supply the **retina** (the light sensitive membrane at the back of the eye) to become blocked or leaky and if left unchecked this can lead to blindness. This is called **diabetic retinopathy**. The human brain and eye compensate very well for gradual loss of vision so you may not be aware that you are developing a problem until it is too late. If you are known to have diabetes and are registered with an NHS GP, you will automatically be called every year for a special eye test. If changes are caught early they can often be treated with laser therapy to prevent things getting worse.

Kidney disease

If the blood supply to your kidneys is affected by diabetes then your kidneys can't work as well. If left unchecked this can lead to kidney failure and would mean you need dialysis or possibly a kidney transplant. Keeping your blood sugar levels well controlled can help prevent this.

Nerve damage

It's not just the big blood vessels that are damaged by high sugar levels, the very tiny vessels that supply your nerves can also be affected and this can lead to a burning sensation known as **neuralgia**. It can also lead to numbness which means you may not feel things normally. If I have a small stone in my shoe it causes me pain; I will take my shoe off and remove the stone. If your nerves have been damaged by diabetes you may not be aware of that stone and so could potentially walk around on it all day. This could lead to an ulcer forming and because of the circulatory problems this may be very difficult to heal in diabetes. If the nerves to the gut are affected it can cause big problems with diarrhoea or constipation.

Foot problems

The combination of nerve damage and poor circulation make you more prone to ulceration and infection. This is one reason why anyone with diabetes is entitled to free podiatry on the NHS and it is well worth getting your feet checked regularly. If you struggle with nail cutting for example, a podiatrist or chiropodist can do this for you to ensure that you don't cut your skin.

Sexual problems

Men with diabetes are more likely to develop erectile dysfunction due to nerve and blood vessel damage. Even if you think this isn't a problem to you emotionally or sexually, you should mention it to your doctor as it could be an indication that you have other circulatory problems that need checking out.

Stillbirth and miscarriage

Women with diabetes who become pregnant tend to have bigger babies and are more likely to miscarry or have a still-birth. Most antenatal care today is provided by midwives in the community but pregnant women with diabetes are likely to be looked after in hospital to minimize any risks.

Travelling with diabetes

Diabetes shouldn't mean you can't travel but it will mean that you have to plan ahead. Delays to your journey could be an issue for you and as meal times may be a little unpredictable, it is worth always carrying carbohydrate snacks with you so that you have control over when you eat. If you are going away for any length of time take a copy of your prescription with you so that you can tell a doctor exactly what you are on in case you should lose your medication. If you are flying, keep your medication with you in hand luggage so that you have it to hand should there be any delays and if you need to use needles ask your doctor for a covering letter explaining why you need to carry them with you to avoid any problems with security.

Pancreatitis

Pancreatitis is inflammation (*itis*) of the pancreas and we distinguish between two types – acute, which causes a short term illness, and chronic, which is associated with irreversible long-term damage to the pancreas.

Who gets pancreatitis?

The most common causes of pancreatitis are gallstones (see Chapter 9) and drinking alcohol excessively, but other risk factors include:

- abdominal injury
- pancreatic tumours

- some viruses, such as mumps or Epstein Barr virus
- cystic fibrosis
- some medications
- high calcium levels in the blood
- high cholesterol.

What are the symptoms of pancreatitis?

Acute pancreatitis causes severe abdominal pain, usually in the upper part of your abdomen and sometimes radiating through to your back. You may also feel and be sick. You will have a high temperature and a rapid pulse. This is a very serious condition and needs urgent medical attention. Chronic pancreatitis is more likely to make you feel very fatigued. You may notice that you pass pale stools, which look oily and tend to float on the water, and you will almost certainly lose weight. Acute pancreatitis can lead to the chronic form.

How is pancreatitis diagnosed and treated?

Pancreatitis is diagnosed following scans and blood tests. Treatment will depend on the severity of your disease. In the acute stages you will be kept nil by mouth to allow your pancreas to recover. You will need drip feeds and painkillers. You will have intravenous antibiotics and may need surgery. If you have had a bout of pancreatitis, you will be advised to avoid alcohol for several months or maybe for ever.

Pancreatic cancer

Pancreatic cancer is the eleventh most common cancer in the UK. Nearly 9,000 people are diagnosed each year.

Who gets pancreatic cancer?

Pancreatic cancer tends to affect older people. It is rare under the age of 40. It affects men and women equally but is more common in smokers, people who drink alcohol to excess, those with diabetes and stomach ulcers, hepatitis and chronic pancreatitis.

What are the symptoms of pancreatic cancer?

One of the main problems with this disease is it often presents late because symptoms don't usually develop until the disease is quite advanced. When they do occur they include stomach or back pain, unexplained weight loss and jaundice.

How is pancreatic cancer diagnosed?

If your GP suspects pancreatic cancer, he or she will arrange blood tests and scans. These may include an ultrasound, CT or MRI. The scans will also help your doctors work out whether the cancer has spread, which will influence treatment.

How is pancreatic cancer treated?

If the cancer has not spread you will be offered surgery with the aim of completely removing the tumour and hope for a cure. This is major surgery and other factors will have to be taken into account such as any other medical conditions you may have and how physically fit you are. Your specialists will discuss all the options with you and you should be involved in the decision-making at all times. Cancer that has spread may require chemotherapy and/or radiotherapy.

10

The liver and gall bladder

Alcohol

Current recommended limits for alcohol in the UK are 14 units a week for women and 21 for men, with at least two alcohol-free days each week. Historically we always referred to a unit as a small glass of wine, half a pint of beer or a single spirit. The problem is a home-poured gin and tonic or glass of wine is likely to be significantly more than a unit so it is easy to exceed recommendations without knowing it.

The simplest way to calculate your units is to look at the percentage alcohol of the drink you are drinking. That is the number of units in a litre of that fluid. So, say you are drinking 12 per cent wine (and many wines are significantly stronger), there will be 12 units in a litre of that fluid. That means there are nine units in a standard 75 cl bottle of wine. A home-poured glass of wine is likely to 250 millilitres, which is three units and the whole bottle is most of your weekly allowance!

Does it matter if I drink more than my recommended units?

Unfortunately it does. Alcohol is toxic to the liver and if you consistently drink above recommended limits you run the risk of developing fatty infiltration of the liver. The problem is that you may not have any symptoms from this, so won't necessarily have any warning signs that you are in trouble. The liver has amazing powers of regeneration and if you stop drinking, a fatty liver will recover completely. If you don't you could go on to develop inflammation of the liver (hepatitis). Again if you stop drinking at this stage, the liver will still recover but, if you don't, you run the risk of developing cirrhosis, which is irreversible and can cause liver failure and liver cancer. There are lots of other medical problems associated with excess alcohol intake and these include:

- gastritis and peptic ulcers (see Chapter 5)
- high blood pressure
- heart failure
- strokes
- erectile dysfunction
- osteoporosis (thin bones)
- dementia
- cancer of the mouth, throat, oesophagus, stomach, colon, liver and breast.

Hepatitis

The term hepatitis simply means inflammation of the liver. Most commonly this is caused by infection or poisoning by alcohol or other drugs.

How would I know if I had hepatitis?

Hepatitis will make you feel fatigued and nauseous. You may also have a fever and a headache. Occasionally, but not always, you will develop a yellow tinge to your skin and the whites of your eyes, which is jaundice.

What causes hepatitis?

There are several types of hepatitis.

- *Hepatitis A* This is the most common form of viral hepatitis. Most cases in the UK are caught during foreign travel and are due to eating contaminated food. When I say contaminated I mean contaminated with faeces from someone who already has the infection so we are talking poor hygiene. If you are going to high risk areas such as Africa, India, Central and South America, the Far East and eastern Europe you can have a vaccine to protect yourself.

- *Hepatitis B* This is passed on via body fluids namely blood, semen and vaginal secretions. It is recommended that health care workers and high risk individuals such as intravenous drug users are vaccinated against Hep B. Most people clear the virus but some individuals develop a chronic form which can lead to cirrhosis and liver cancer.
- *Hepatitis C* This is most commonly spread through blood contact and three-quarters of sufferers will go on to have the chronic form which is associated with cirrhosis and liver cancer. There is, as yet, no available vaccine for Hep C.
- *Hepatitis D* This is only seen in conjunction with Hepatitis B.
- *Hepatitis E* This is extremely rare in the UK.
- *Alcoholic hepatitis* As many as one in four heavy drinkers will develop this.
- *Autoimmune hepatitis* This is more common in women than men and is caused by the body developing antibodies to its own liver.

Cirrhosis

Cirrhosis is the term used when normal healthy liver tissue has been replaced by scar tissue. It is irreversible and can lead to liver failure and liver cancer. There are 30,000 people in the UK today with cirrhotic livers. It can be caused by a number of different conditions including:

- excess alcohol consumption, one in ten heavy drinkers will eventually develop cirrhosis;
- chronic hepatitis B and C;
- autoimmune hepatitis;
- some medications;
- heart failure;
- haemochromatosis, a condition where iron accumulates in the body;

- Wilson's disease, a condition where copper accumulates in the body.

How would I know if I had cirrhosis?

Cirrhosis will make you feel fatigued and weak. You are likely to lose your appetite and feel or be sick. You may notice a yellow tinge to your skin and the whites of your eyes and the build up of this pigment may make you feel very itchy. You are likely to bruise more easily as your liver struggles, because many of the clotting factors are made in the liver. You may develop a swollen abdomen and you may become mentally confused, or change your personality as the liver is unable to clear toxins, which then build up in your brain.

How is cirrhosis diagnosed?

Liver blood tests may show that the liver is under strain but cirrhosis is confirmed on an ultrasound test.

How is cirrhosis treated?

Treatment involves treating the underlying cause and whatever the cause, even if it has nothing to do with alcohol, it is important that you stop drinking alcohol altogether as your liver is already compromised and it doesn't need any more insults. You may need water pills (**diuretics**) to reduce the fluid retention and swelling and you will be advised to stick to a low salt diet. You may be give tablets to reduce your itching. Since cirrhosis is irreversible the only cure is a liver transplant.

Gallstones

Gallstones are made by an imbalance of cholesterol and bile pigments in the gall bladder.

Who gets gallstones?

When I was at medical school we were taught that gallstones were found in the 'fair, fat and forty', in other words, in overweight middle-aged women and certainly they are three times more common in women than in men, and they are more common in older people. Obesity is a well-recognized risk factor. Other risk factors include:

- having a relative with gallstones
- rapid weight loss
- pregnancy
- hormone replacement therapy
- Crohn's disease.

How would I know if I had gallstones?

You might not! Most people with gallstones don't have any symptoms but if they do cause problems, you will develop severe upper right sided abdominal pain. You will feel and may be sick and you will develop a temperature. This presentation is called **cholecystitis**.

How are gallstones diagnosed?

Gallstones are diagnosed using an abdominal ultrasound.

How are gallstones treated?

If your gallstones are not causing symptoms you and your doctor may choose to leave things be, but if you have had an attack of cholecystitis and certainly if you are getting recurrent attacks your doctor will recommend that you have your gall bladder removed. This can usually be done with keyhole surgery (laparoscopy). If your gall bladder is removed laparoscopically, you should be back to normal within a couple of weeks but open surgery will take about six weeks for a full recovery.

11

Food allergy and intolerance

The subject of allergy probably warrants a book to itself but I wanted to include a brief chapter on this in digestive health because I see so much confusion in my surgery about the difference between food allergies and intolerances, and I think it's important that we understand the difference. I have often heard people refer to an intolerance as a 'mild allergy', which is not the case. The two conditions are very different.

Food allergy

A food allergy is where the body identifies a certain food as harmful and develops antibodies to it. These IgE antibodies trigger an immune reaction, causing the release of histamine and other allergenic chemicals. Typical symptoms of an IgE-mediated allergy include a skin rash called **urticaria**. This looks like nettle rash and is intensely itchy. Patients may feel very unwell with diarrhoea and vomiting, their lips and tongue may swell and they become wheezy. This is a medical emergency and if not treated urgently can be fatal. It is called **anaphylactic shock**.

We can do blood tests to look for specific antibodies to particular foods and anyone with a confirmed allergy like this will need to carry an adrenalin pen for injection should they inadvertently be exposed to that food. We can develop an allergy to any food but 90 per cent of food allergies in the UK are due to:

- wheat, rye, barley and oats
- shellfish

- eggs
- fish
- oysters and mussels
- nuts
- sesame seeds
- soya.

The important thing to remember here is that food allergies develop very quickly, often within minutes of exposure and even trace amounts of a food can trigger an anaphylactic reaction, which is why you so often hear an announcement on a plane, for example, that no one must eat any peanuts. It is possible to have a partial allergy. By that I mean some people can tolerate a food if it is well cooked but not in its raw state, so a child with an allergy to eggs may be able to eat a cake made with eggs which has been baked, but would develop symptoms if exposed to mayonnaise made with raw eggs. The reverse can also be true; for example, celery and celeriac seem to be more allergenic when cooked.

Generally speaking once an allergy has developed it is with you for life. Young children who are allergic to eggs, milk, wheat or soya, however, will often grow out of their allergies by the age of five. Only consider reintroducing a food that has previously caused an allergic reaction in consultation with your doctor. Allergies to nuts, shellfish and fish are very rarely lost, and if you have an allergy to one food you are at increased risk of developing an allergy to another one. If you have a true allergy to a food, you will need to cut it out of your diet and may need to see a dietician to ensure that you are replacing any lost nutrients with other foods.

Food intolerance

Food intolerances are less clear cut. The symptoms may be more vague and the time frames are often less obvious. A food intolerance will not produce IgE antibodies to that food.

Symptoms often take hours or even days to occur so it can take a long while before the diagnosis is made. Common symptoms include abdominal pain, bloating, diarrhoea or constipation. Patients often describe a feeling of lethargy and poor concentration. Intolerances may occur because of a difficulty digesting a particular food. This can be because of low levels of an enzyme required to break down that food, such as lactase needed to break down lactose, the natural sugar occurring in milk. It is also possible to be intolerant to chemicals in foods such as caffeine, monosodium glutamate and salicylates.

Unlike allergies, some people find that they can tolerate small amounts of a particular food but develop symptoms if they over-indulge. We can't do blood tests for intolerances and I find the best way to identify an intolerance is to keep a detailed food and symptom diary to see if there is a link between diet and symptoms. If there appears to be a link, try cutting out that food while still keeping a symptom diary and, hopefully, things will become clearer.

Intolerances, unlike allergies, may be transient, so you may be able to tolerate a given food at some point in the future.

Index